THE
ROAD
CYCLING
PERFORMANCE MANUAL

BLOOMSBURY SPORT
Bloomsbury Publishing Plc
50 Bedford Square, London, WC1B 3DP, UK

BLOOMSBURY, BLOOMSBURY SPORT
and the Diana logo are trademarks of
Bloomsbury Publishing Plc

First published in Great Britain 2018

Copyright © Nikalas Cook, 2018
Photos © Getty Images, 2018
Photo research by Adrian Besley
With special thanks to Alex Davis

Bloomsbury Publishing Plc does not have
any control over, or responsibility for, any
third-party websites referred to or in this
book. All internet addresses given in this book
were correct at the time of going to press. The
author and publisher regret any inconvenience
caused if addresses have changed or sites
have ceased to exist, but can accept no
responsibility for any such changes

A catalogue record for this book is available
from the British Library

Library of Congress Cataloging-in-Publication
data has been applied for

ISBN: PB: 978-1-4729-4444-3
        eBook: 978-1-4729-4445-0

2 4 6 8 10 9 7 5 3 1

Designed by Austin Taylor
Printed and bound in China by
C&C Offset Printing Co.

Bloomsbury Publishing Plc makes every
effort to ensure that the papers used in
the manufacture of our books are natural,
recyclable products made from wood grown
in well-managed forests. Our manufacturing
processes conform to the environmental
regulations of the country of origin.

To find out more about our authors and books
visit www.bloomsbury.com and sign up for our
newsletters

We recognise that the following terms:
TrainingPeaks, Training Stress Score (TSS),
Performance Management Chart (PMC),
Acute Training Load (ATL), Chronic Training
Load (CTL), Training Stress Balance (TSB),
are all registered copyright ®

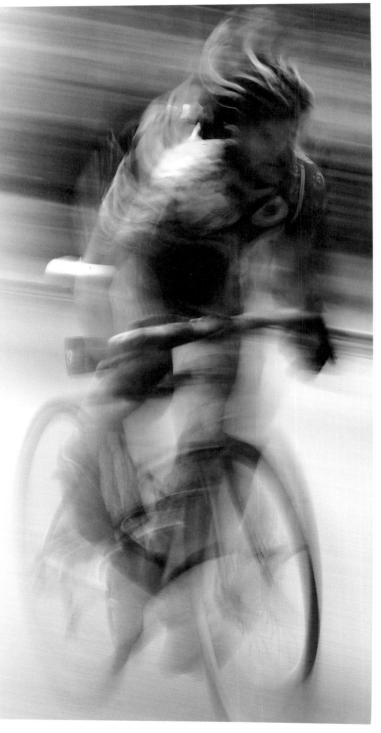

NIKALAS COOK

THE ROAD CYCLING
PERFORMANCE MANUAL

EVERYTHING YOU NEED TO TAKE YOUR TRAINING AND RACING TO THE NEXT LEVEL

BLOOMSBURY SPORT
LONDON · OXFORD · NEW YORK · NEW DELHI · SYDNEY

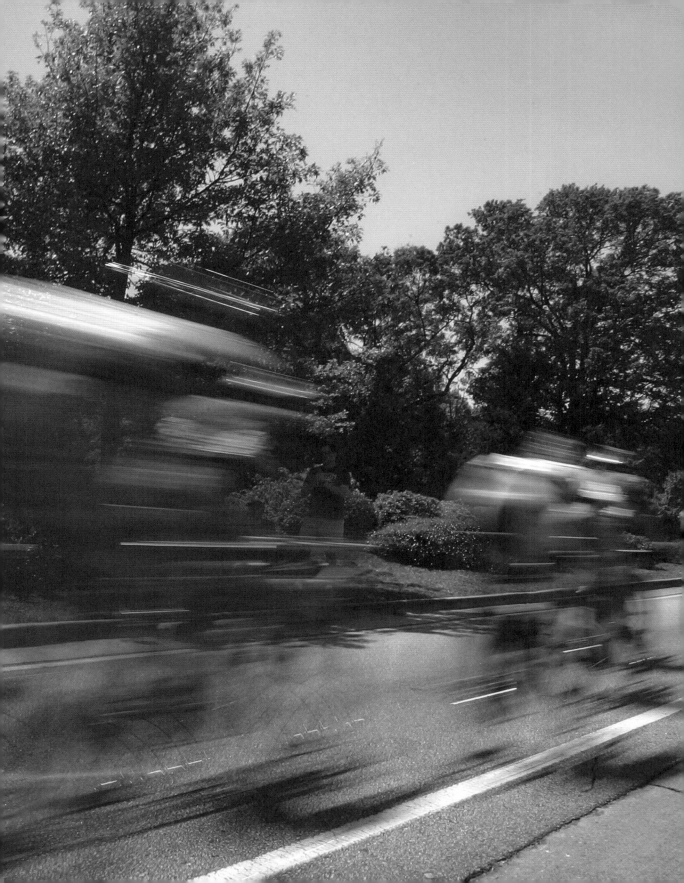

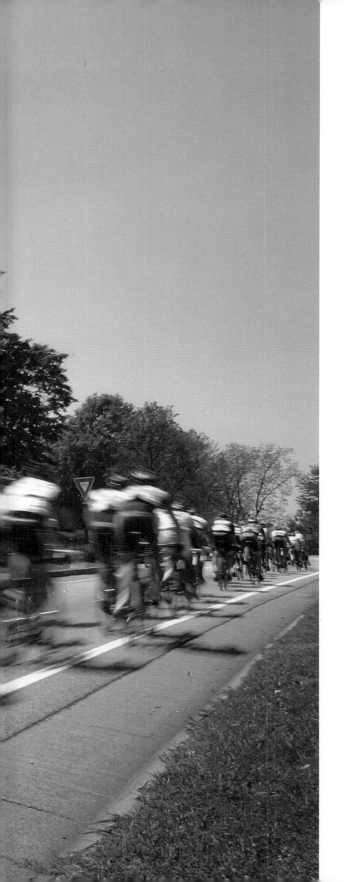

CONTENTS

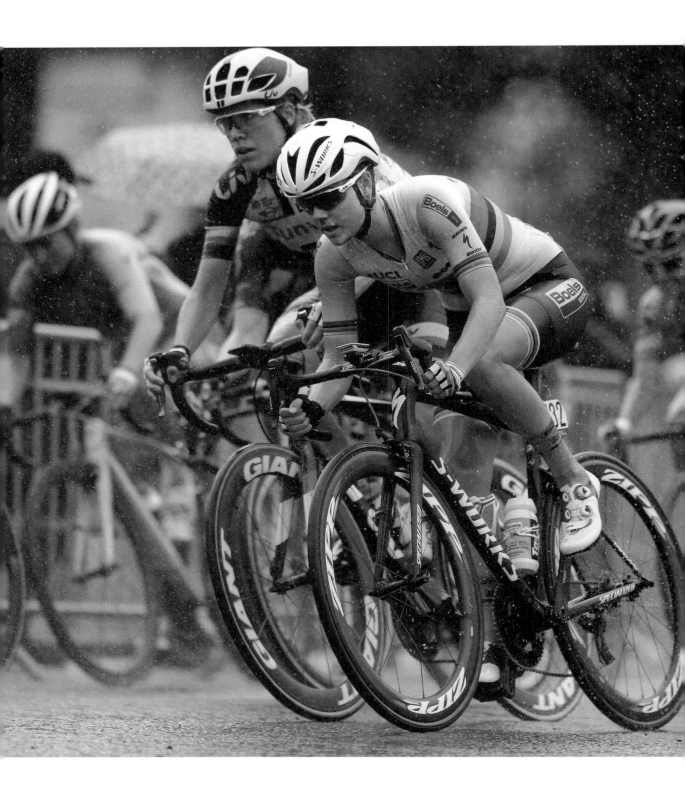

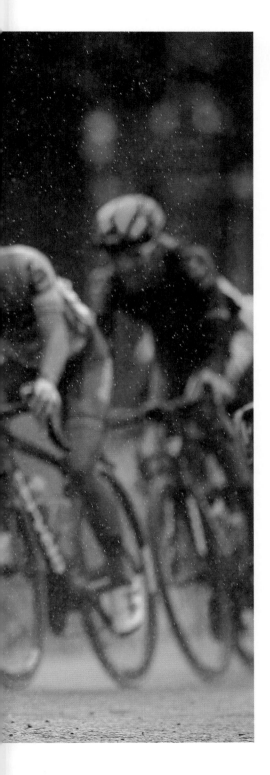

FOREWORD

ALTHOUGH THE GREAT BRITISH Cycling Team is synonymous with the aggregation of marginal gains and leaving no stone unturned in the search for those 100th of seconds that can decide a gold medal, this focusing on the minutiae can only work if all the fundamentals are in place first. Although the top secret high-tech kit receives the bulk of media attention, having worked with the team through three Olympic cycles, it's getting the basics 100% right, whether it's training, kit, bike set-up or nutrition, that lays the foundations of success.

This approach of ensuring that all of the key aspects of performance are addressed first is at the heart of Nik's training philosophy. It's especially relevant to time starved cyclists who want to maximise the gains available from their limited training time. If you're out on the bike, in the gym or looking to spend some of your hard earned cash, it's by applying the fundamentals first that give you the best bang for your buck.

I first met Nik producing training plans and supporting content together for British Cycling and found him to have an excellent knowledge and understanding of the sport. He has a great ability to take complex and technical information and convey it in an accessible manner. However, it was after suffering a severe injury, a ruptured patella tendon, that I really saw both his drive and his application of his training methods to himself.

Having guided him through a lengthy rehabilitation process, taking four months to be able to complete a single pedal rotation on a static bike, and getting him back out on the road, he set himself the ambitious target of competing at the Masters World Track Championships. To not only take part but to win gold in the Team Pursuit, setting a World's Best Time, is testament to both his ability as a rider and his knowledge in designing and implementing a training plan to take himself to that point.

I've no doubt that, if you're looking to improve your own performance on the bike, following Nik's advice and applying his training philosophy to your own riding will definitely help you to achieve your personal goals on the bike.

PHIL BURT, FORMER LEAD PHYSIOTHERAPIST WITH THE
GREAT BRITAIN CYCLING TEAM

INTRODUCTION

THE AIM OF THIS BOOK is to help you take your road cycling to the next level. Whether you're looking to improve your performance at your next sportive, beat your time trial best, topple a Strava King of the Mountain (KOM) or move up a racing category, the fundamental knowledge provided here will help you to achieve your goal. Road cycling is a wonderful sport that allows you to ride on the same roads as your heroes and heroines, and, with the advent of GPS and social media, even compare your performances. In this book, we look at the techniques used by top riders and teams, and then adapt and utilise this information, applying it in a realistic and attainable way to your riding.

The Road Performance Cycling Manual provides a comprehensive training guide from which you'll be able to construct your own training plan and target it towards your key events. The book draws on the expertise of some of the best nutritionists, physiotherapists and coaches in cycling but distils their knowledge in a practical and applicable way. I'll pass on the little gems of knowledge and tips that I've learned over the years, and you'll find practical and easy-to-follow advice on everything from bike set-up, must-own kit and equipment to how to make those final days before a big event go smoothly.

Minimising maximal losses

Cycling had long been a sport whose training methods were largely based on little more than hearsay and tradition rather than solid sports science. Even at the highest levels of the sport, ex-riders retired, became coaches and, without questioning them, passed on the rituals and traditions to the next generation. Whether it was tucking into a steak before a race, grinding out seemingly endless slow miles during the winter or never considering any 'off the bike' training, that was how it had always been done. It genuinely took a revolution to break this cycle of misinformation, and the epicentre of that revolution was the National Cycling Centre in Manchester, England.

There's no disputing the fact that, since 2008 and the Beijing Olympics, Britain has established itself as the world's number one cycling nation, with the Great Britain Cycling Team taking medal hauls at the Beijing, London and Rio Olympics that made other nations green with envy and Team Sky racking up multiple Grand Tour wins. One of the most publicised reasons for this success has been their philosophy of the aggregation of marginal gains. This entails looking at every aspect of cycling, such as kit, nutrition, training methods, recovery and health, and optimising them all. The improvements from just one of these areas may be small but, by adding up lots of small gains, they become significant. The infamous Secret Squirrel Club at British Cycling, headed by Chris Boardman, left no stone unturned in their hunt for gains, even producing exact replicas

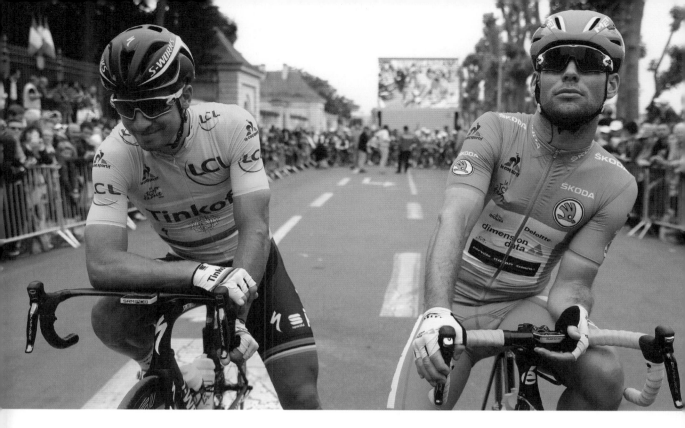

of riders for wind tunnel testing and producing a skinsuit so effective that the UCI ended up banning it. In a sport deeply rooted in tradition, some of these ideas were initially met with scorn and even ridicule, especially when Team Sky took this philosophy into the ultra-conservative world of road racing. They lugged their own mattresses and pillows from hotel to hotel on Grand Tours to ensure that their riders got the best night's sleep possible, and even experimented with their team leaders using a motorhome. After a hard mountaintop finish, rather than getting straight into the team bus, they'd cool down on turbos. And as other teams and nations saw the results that Sky and British Cycling were achieving, the laughter stopped and the imitating started.

There's no doubt that for professional cyclists and Olympians, this accumulation of marginal gains approach is incredibly effective and important. The main reason for this is that all the basics of their training, nutrition and equipment are spot on and the way for them to find that extra 1 per cent, which can make the difference between winning and losing, is to dial in on the detail. However, for the vast majority of riders, these fundamental boxes simply aren't being properly ticked. They get distracted and confused analysing the minutiae of their cycling, ignore the key basics and fail to reach their full potential.

This is why I like to think in terms of minimising maximal losses. It's about avoiding the common mistakes, getting the fundamentals right and maximising your potential. There are four main areas to consider:

1 Your bike set-up, equipment and clothing should aid you, not inhibit you from achieving your training or event goals. A slammed stem may look cool and pro but if it means you're having to stop and stretch your back every ten minutes, you're not going to set many personal bests. Similarly, if you're too cold or too hot, your body will be wasting valuable energy that could be going into your pedals. Also, how many riders have you seen at a time trial with all the latest go-faster aero kit, only to pin their number on so it acts like a parachute and in one stroke negate all the gains their kit is giving them? Don't worry, I'm not going to be a kit killjoy (I like a shiny bit of carbon as much as the next rider) but, by getting the basics right, you'll get more value out of your pricey upgrades.

2 Training has to be consistent, structured, progressive and driven by your goals, strengths and weaknesses. Many riders make the mistake of thinking that more is more and fail to prioritise recovery. This means you just become more fatigued rather than gaining fitness. It's only by allowing your body to recover from training that it adapts and becomes stronger. You have to allow adequate recovery between tough training sessions, schedule regular recovery weeks into your training and ensure that you taper down to important events. Progression is essential to give your body new stimuli to adapt to. How many riders do you know that do exactly the same routine, week in, week out? Evolution has hardwired our bodies to be fundamentally lazy; unless you give them good reason to change, they won't. Intensity has to be monitored, whether using a heart rate monitor, a power meter or a combination of both. Without doing this, you're training blind. I've heard some riders make the argument that using these training tools is taking things too seriously and is only really for the pros. This couldn't be further from the truth. With

limited time to train, ensuring that you're getting the most out of every pedal stroke is a no-brainer. Monitoring intensity allows you to achieve this. Constructing a training plan isn't rocket science and certainly isn't the dark art that some coaches make it out to be, and in this book you will be given all the tools and information you need to formulate your own training plan and tailor it to your personal goals.

3 Nutrition is another key area, both on and off the bike. Unfortunately, more than any other area of sports performance, there's a bewildering amount of misinformation and poor science associated with nutrition. Knowing how to correctly fuel and hydrate before, during and after your rides is crucial, but a huge number of riders get it massively wrong. Off the bike, fad diets promising weight loss and improved performance only add to the confusion. Certainly, for many riders, losing a few pounds definitely comes under the umbrella of minimising maximal losses, but it has to be done safely, sensibly and sustainably. Some supplements can legally boost your performance, but there's little point using these expensive products, which will give limited gains at best, unless you're getting your nutritional basics right.

4 Pacing, whether you're out for a training ride, taking part in a sportive or racing in a time trial, is the factor that can really make or break a ride. Learning to pace optimally begins with testing for your threshold heart rate or power, and you'll come to see this number as your cycling 'red line', using it to set accurate heart rate or power zones and then practise, practise and practise. It's then about having the discipline, even when you pin a number on, to stick to your tried and tested pacing strategy. Pacing is also intrinsically linked to fuelling. If you're going too hard, your body won't be able to digest the food you're giving it. The food you try to take on will just sit in your stomach, making you feel bloated and nauseous.

Not a full-time cyclist

ALTHOUGH THERE'S NO DISPUTING the fact that professional cyclists are probably the hardest working and toughest sportspeople on the planet, as non-professional cyclists, in some ways, we have it tougher. You have to fit your training around work, family and other commitments. You probably don't get to spend hours lounging on the sofa after a hard ride – after all, that lawn won't mow itself. You definitely don't have a team car following you on your training rides and I'm guessing that a massage is an occasional treat rather than a daily norm. This is why, although we can learn from what the pros do, it's imperative not to try to copy them exactly.

One of the main reasons for this is the physical and mental stress that daily life puts on our bodies. Pro cyclists are masters of doing nothing when not riding. When not training they'll be horizontal, avoiding being on their feet whenever possible and always taking lifts rather than using stairs. This lifestyle allows their bodies to cope with and adapt to the immense training and racing volume that they are subjected to. Their only training stress is the training that they're doing. We have to factor in additional stresses other than our training. If it's a really busy period at work, you've got a new-born baby or you're undertaking a big home improvement project, it's probably not the time to inflict a hard training block on yourself. A coach friend of mine told me a great example of this. He was coaching a rider who, according to his training diary, was completing every session, but the problem was that his performance was mysteriously dropping. It transpired that, due to being under heavy work pressure, he'd been getting up before dawn every morning to fit in his workout ahead of a 12-hour-plus working day. He was hammering himself into the ground, forgetting that scheduling in and completing adequate recovery is as important as nailing every workout.

Another case of not following the lead of the pros is winter training. Traditional winter base training involves going out and riding at a steady pace for hours on end. The rationale for this is to build a solid base of endurance fitness, develop efficiency and the body's ability to burn fat as a fuel, and prepare for the higher-intensity training as the rider transitions into the racing season. This approach to winter training works well for the pros, as they're able to devote the necessary 30–35 hours of riding a week to it. They get their training stimulus from this base work because of the volume of work they're doing. If you're only able to ride for six to ten hours a week, there's very little point in doing them all slowly. I'm not saying that there's no place for endurance-focused rides – far from it – and they're key to cycling success, but you also have to include some higher-intensity work to maximise your winter gains.

I hope you take a lot from this book, find it interesting and informative and, more than anything, find that it improves your cycling performance.

Enjoy the ride.

Nikalas Cook

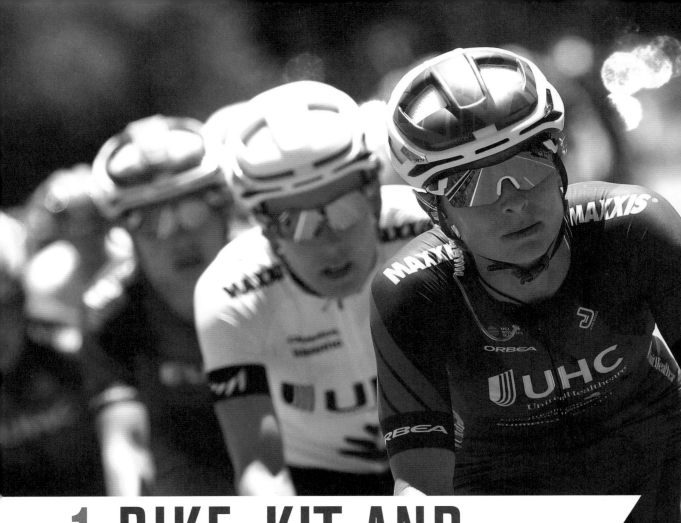

1 BIKE, KIT AND EQUIPMENT

THERE'S NOTHING WRONG WITH TREATING YOURSELF TO SOME BLING NEW CYCLING KIT BUT WHAT SHOULD YOU BE SPENDING YOUR MONEY ON TO MAKE THE BIGGEST DIFFERENCE TO YOUR CYCLING?

'Don't buy upgrades; ride up grades.' EDDY MERCKX

IF WE'RE ALL BEING HONEST with ourselves, one of the main appeals of cycling is the bike and its accompanying kit. We're all guilty of constantly thinking about that next bike, go-faster wheelset or must-have high-tech and high-performing item of clothing. There's absolutely nothing wrong with this, it's part of the fun, and if you can afford the best kit, I don't see why you shouldn't treat yourself to it, regardless of your riding ability. Don't be put off by 'all the gear, no idea' mockery and inverse snobbery; if having great kit makes you feel good and motivates you to ride, go for it. However, it's not the bike and the kit that makes a successful cyclist, and cycling doesn't have to be a cripplingly expensive pastime. If you're reading this book, you're looking to improve your cycling and shouldn't need your hand held through the process of buying

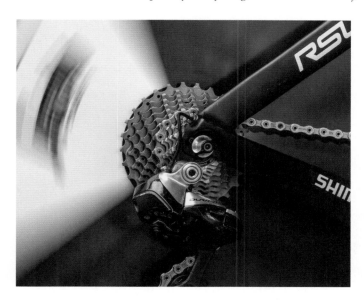

▲ A shiny top end of the range groupset may be a tempting upgrade but probably won't be the best investment in terms of performance gains.

a bike. Prioritise getting the best frame you can, even if that means dropping a groupset level or two, as you can always upgrade components down the line but it's the heart of the bike that makes the real difference. If possible, get a fit done before buying to establish the geometry and frame size you need and use that information to inform your decision. You probably already have strong opinions on frame materials, Shimano versus Campagnolo versus SRAM, and your preferred brand of bib shorts, so I'm not going to cover those basics, aside from a brief comment about frame materials. Whether it's carbon, alloy (aluminium), steel or titanium, a poor-quality frame is poor quality. By the same token, if you go for a reputable brand, regardless of material used, it'll perform. In the professional peloton, there's no denying that carbon is now king and, for its strength and stiffness-to-weight ratio, ease of moulding to aero profiles and affordability, it's easy to see why. However, a pro team requires a staggering number of bikes and has to kowtow to sponsors. This makes the use of bespoke and artisan steel and titanium unrealistic, but for non-pros looking for that one-off dream bike, you won't necessarily be limiting yourself by not choosing carbon. Don't worry about the supposed fragility or limited shelf life of carbon, this is largely a myth. It's an incredibly strong and resilient material that stands up, not only to the power put out by the likes of Sir Chris Hoy or Kristina Vogel in a sprint, but also the stresses generated by a Formula 1 car or a jet aircraft. It's also not prone to the accumulation of fatigue that metals suffer from so, in theory, if well looked after, should outlast a metal frame. Carbon is extremely strong in the direction that it's designed to take load in but can be relatively fragile to impact and crushing. Classics are handlebars spinning round into the top-tube, damage from over-tightening components or crushing in a work stand. Invest in and learn to use a torque wrench, use carbon assembly paste to reduce the amount of torque required and always be mindful of not applying crushing or impact forces. If your carbon frame does get damaged, it's not the end as there are a number of companies now offering excellent repair services. Look after it well and a carbon frame can last you a lifetime.

What I will deal with in this chapter are the 'biggest bang for your buck' things that you can spend your hard-earned money on. The items that'll give you the biggest return on your investment and allow you to train and ride to your maximum potential. These include ensuring that your bike fits properly, and overcoming the complaint of every cyclist, from novice to pro, of saddle soreness. I'll also address buying and setting up an

'I see it all the time: an obviously fit cyclist using a good bike, but riding in a position so bad that it cancels out most of the advantages of the expensive machine and the hours of training.' **PHIL BURT**, FORMER LEAD PHYSIOTHERAPIST WITH THE GREAT BRITAIN CYCLING TEAM

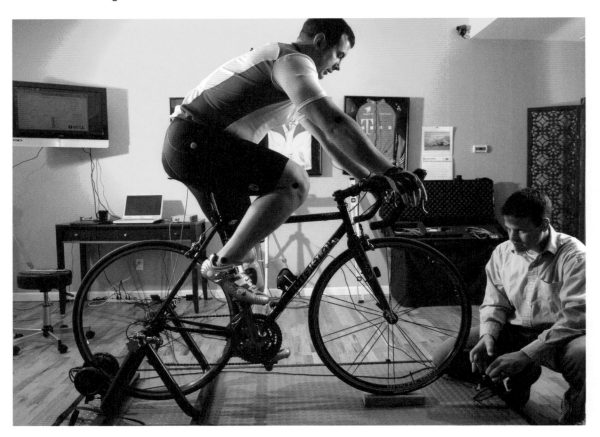

indoor trainer, and why using one isn't just about not riding in the rain. If you don't already own one, I'll explain why buying and learning to use a power meter is probably the best investment you can make. Finally, if you're looking at adding a bike to your stable, I'll advise about which type will have the greatest benefit to your overall riding.

Professional bike fit

Apart from the delectable searing pain in your legs when you push hard, there's no reason to suffer pain or discomfort on the bike. Whether it's lower back stiffness, numbness in your hands or feet, or sore knees, there's no need for it. A combination of a professional bike fit and maybe some prescribed off the bike conditioning work should make cycling pain free, until you want it to hurt. Getting a professional bike fit, especially if you do suffer from discomfort or have a history of injury, is a no-brainer investment. If you can keep pedalling strongly for four or five hours, without having to constantly squirm in your saddle or stop to stretch out your back, the gains over a long sportive will be measurable in minutes, definitely not a marginal gain. If a bike fit prevents you picking up an overuse injury or compounding an existing one, you'll be saving yourself an enforced layoff from riding and possibly the cost of physiotherapist bills.

◄ If you're spending thousands on a bike, investing a couple of hundred on a professional bike fit is a no-brainer

Bike fits have become increasingly available to all riders, but how do you know you're getting a good one and what should you look for?

THE TRADITIONAL BIKE FIT METHOD In a really old school traditional bike shop, you might be sized up for a frame and given a position based on the Italian CONI bike-fitting manual. Published in 1972, it looked at a group of 20-year-old professional cyclists and, because they rode fast, assumed that the commonalities of their positions would make everyone ride fast. Unfortunately, this doesn't hold true and although it's a quick and easy method, it won't take any account of your individual body type and it forces your body to adapt to the bike.

OBSERVATIONAL BIKE FITS Observational fits based on the beliefs of the fitter of what a rider's position should look like. You'll often find this style of fitting in bike shops and, sitting on a jig and listening to the sage-like words of the fitter, it can seem very convincing. It's an improvement on a traditional CONI fit as it does at least look at the individual, but with no objective data and relying on the fitter's take on a good position, most riders end up looking the same.

OBJECTIVE DATA BIKE FITS You've then got a host of generic formulae and equations, based on measurements such as inseam, that are used to predict saddle heights and other components of fit. This style of fitting does at least gather some objective data and recognises that proportions are important to bike fitting, but it fails because it's totally static, generic and doesn't even consider how the rider interacts with their bike.

STATIC BIKE FITS With a static individualised fit, it's heading in the right direction and starting to utilise methodical and repeatable techniques. You'll sit on a jig and, using a plumb bob and goniometer, the fitter will use accepted ranges of joint angles to optimise fit. The problem is that cycling isn't a static activity and an apparently ideal position on the jig can fall apart once the rider starts to pedal.

DYNAMIC BIKE FITS Moving into the 21st century, dynamic fits can be conducted using video analysis and motion capture. Retül and Dartfish are both examples of this type of fit. Although it's more costly than the other methods, this is the gold standard for getting an accurate and personalised bike fit. However, motion capture isn't instant bike-fitting nirvana. Even with the best kit, a fit is only as good as the experience and knowledge of the fitter conducting it. Too many fitters are simply applying neutral ranges without considering and accommodating the unique qualities of the rider. This is where doing some research really counts and I'd strongly recommend finding a fitting studio that offers a physiotherapist-led bike fit.

The bike fit process

Before you go anywhere near a jig or motion capture system, the fitter should take a full and detailed history from you. This should include your cycling goals, any problems you currently have and your injury history. Your goals are especially important. For most sportive riders, the number one priority of a fit is comfort or sustainability. However, if you're a time trialist or looking to race shorter duration events on the road or track, comfort is less of an issue and aerodynamics become more important.

The fitter should then move on to a physical examination, assessing your flexibility, mobility and any other factors that might influence your position on the bike. This information, combined with the data collected during the actual bike fit, will allow the

'Bike fit for me is one of the most important factors for success on a bike. If you're not at one with your bike it can create so many problems from not having the power to push the pedals optimally or maybe it's a case of you getting injuries. You see so many people that aren't sitting properly on their bike. Whenever you get a new bike, make sure you get a good bike fit. At our training camp in December we have the opportunity for having our positions checked and this is especially important for new riders who may have been riding a different brand of bike. I don't spend a huge amount of time doing it because I've been riding that long and my position has developed over the years to be pretty efficient. That's important too as, with time, your position will evolve so it's an ongoing process.' **TIFFANY CROMWELL**, CANYON/SRAM

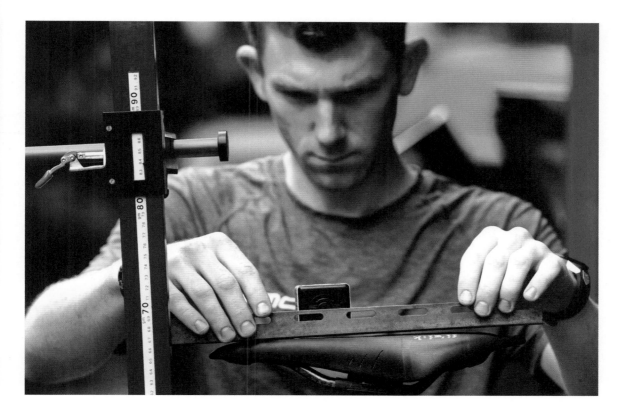

▲ The position you get at the end of a bike fit is only the start of the process of finding your optimal set-up.

fitter to find a suitable riding position for you. This may involve you having to change some components on your bike, such as the stem, saddle, cranks or handlebars, or even potentially finding that your frame just isn't suited to you. For this reason, I'd factor a physio-led bike fit into your budget when buying a new bike. A 3D motion capture system such as Retül can point you towards the frames most suited to accommodate your riding position. By dropping a groupset on your spec or choosing slightly less bling wheels, you'll be able to afford one, and it'll definitely have a far more positive impact on your cycling.

Establishing your position isn't the end of the process, as finding your ideal set-up is a constant evolution. It's likely that you've had to make some compromises, such as sacrificing aerodynamics for comfort or sustainability. You will probably have been given some exercises to help your body adapt to the new position and to allow your position to be further improved in the future.

If you want to find out more about bike fit before committing to one, *Bike Fit: Optimise Your Bike Position for High Performance and Injury Avoidance* by Phil Burt is regarded as the best book on the subject. Phil was the lead physiotherapist for the Great Britain Cycling Team and, as well as being one of the leading minds in bike fitting, is an unsung hero of the last three Olympic Games. His knowledge and experience is unparalleled and I'd consider his book a must-have for your cycling library.

The madness of crank length

One aspect of your bike fit, especially if you're shorter in stature, is crank length. Forming the link from your pedals to the drivetrain, your cranks have a direct impact on your saddle height and pedalling dynamics. Many riders will notice a change in saddle height of just a few millimetres, but won't even question their crank length, which can easily vary by up to 10mm (⅜in). If you've bought an off-the-peg bike, chances are its cranks will sit in the fairly limited range of 170–175mm (6⅔–7in) but, even more likely, they'll be the industry bog standard 172.5mm (6¾in). It's not uncommon to find the same 172.5mm cranks fitted to both a 58cm (23in) and a 52cm (20½in) frame. It's only when you get down to small female-specific frames that crank lengths suddenly shrink to 165mm (6½in).

If you assume that the prevalent 172.5mm cranks are aimed at, and are correct for, an average-sized male rider of 5ft 10in (1.78m), you can calculate that your cranks should equate to approximately 9.7 per cent of your height. This is only a rough calculation and there are a number of more sophisticated versions using inside seam length and other variables, but the key fact that these calculations show is that suitable crank length varies significantly more than most bike manufacturers allow for.

This is especially pertinent for shorter riders and if you're less than 5ft 10in, it's very likely that you're currently riding cranks that are too long. If your cranks are too long, in order to be able to adequately extend your knee at the bottom of your pedal stoke, you have to drop your saddle height. When you come to the top of your pedal stroke, this lower saddle height, in combination with the long cranks, means more knee flexion, the associated greater strain on your knees and reduced efficiency.

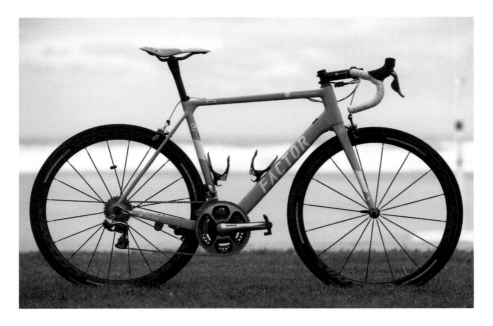

◄ If you're at the tall or small end of the height spectrum and have bought an off the peg bike, check your crank length.

A further knock-on effect is that your angle of hip flexion will be significantly reduced. An overly tight hip angle will result in discomfort and lower power output. You may also experience a sensation of almost kneeing yourself in the chest, especially when down on the drops or in time trial position. Many riders will also find that their hips rotate externally to compensate for this, resulting in a knees-out pedalling style.

It's not unusual when riders do fit correctly sized cranks, especially if they're shorter in stature, to find it has a massive positive impact on their comfort and performance on the bike. Pedalling style can improve, existing knee discomfort can diminish (and even cease), and holding a more aerodynamic position can suddenly become far easier.

Saddle choice and avoiding saddle soreness

As we've already seen, there's no need to be uncomfortable on the bike, and this of course applies to your backside. Even experienced cyclists suffer in silence with saddle soreness or aren't aware of the simple steps they can take to prevent it. After the 2012 Olympic Games, the Great Britain Cycling Team suspected that saddle soreness might be an issue, especially for the female riders, and they conducted a survey. They found that 100 per cent of the riders had suffered from issues, but had just accepted them as part and parcel of cycling. Solving this problem was made a priority and a panel of experts was assembled, including tribologists (friction experts), reconstructive surgeons who were experts in dealing with pressure sores, and top consultants in vulval health. Now all riders on the team are instructed in personal care to minimise soreness, and saddle and chamois technology is constantly being developed. After the Rio Olympics, Laura Kenny was quoted as saying how the work of the medical team with regard to dealing with saddle soreness had changed her life.

Finding the right saddle for you is essential and, although pressure mapping technology and measuring sit bone width can point you in the right direction, it's largely a case of trial and error. If your saddle doesn't feel right, change it. Many shops offer 'try before you buy' — and you should be prepared to try a few before you find one that's right. Don't think that wide and padded necessarily means comfortable and don't be scared of trying some of the more outlandish split-nosed designs. Once you find a saddle that works for you, stick with it and fit the same one on all your bikes.

'Pros often don't get much choice about saddles as you're supposed to ride whatever the sponsors supply. But, when I was with Rapha/Condor/Sharp, we had Fizik, which I really liked. They offered 3 or 4 different saddles based on rider biomechanics and having that choice was brilliant. It makes sense, we're all different and a 60kg five foot nothing climber is bound to want something different to a burly six foot 75kg sprinter.'

DEAN DOWNING, EX-PRO, FORMER BRITISH CIRCUIT RACE CHAMPION AND NOW COACH

Be aware that, in addition to your saddle, your shorts and chamois can have a massive impact on comfort. Seam position and pad shape varies massively between brands and models so, again, you may need to try a few before you find the one that works for you. Don't buy cheap cycling shorts. Budget shorts are a guaranteed route to a sore behind. You may pay more for the recognised and respected manufacturers, but the quality of the pad and the improved comfort it'll deliver will definitely repay your investment.

Once you've found the correct saddle and shorts, make sure you work through the points below to make saddle soreness a thing of the past.

How to avoid saddle soreness

Bike fit Persistent saddle soreness can be a sign that your position on the bike isn't right. If you tend to get sore only on one side, this can be indicative of a possible asymmetry such as a leg length discrepancy.

Chamois cream If you're not using chamois cream, start now. It can feel a bit strange when you first set off if you're not used to it but it does make a big difference.

No knickers Never wear an additional layer between the chamois and your skin. Cotton especially prevents the technical fabrics in the chamois and shorts functioning properly and will trap a layer of moisture next to the skin. This will increase friction and the risk of bacterial infection.

Stand up Even on flat rides, try to stand up out of your saddle every 10–15 minutes to give your backside a bit of a break and to restore some blood flow.

Get your shorts off Don't sit around in your shorts at the end of a ride, get them off and shower as soon as possible. Never, ever reuse a dirty pair of shorts.

Clean and dry When showering, the aim is to get clean but not sterile. Don't scrub, and avoid using flannels, sponges and exfoliators. Avoid removing all the natural oils and bacteria, both of which enhance the barrier function of the epidermis. Use a gentle washing cream, such as Dermol 500, and always rinse well with plenty of plain water. Pat dry and avoid rubbing. Wear loose clothing to aid drying and airflow. You can also use an unperfumed moisturiser to improve barrier function.

Keep it natural down there Mainly for the ladies, but I know some male riders also like the trimmed option. Pubic hair helps with the transport and evaporation of sweat away from the skin. It also provides some friction protection. Hair removal methods, such as shaving, depilatory creams and epilation, are damaging to the epidermis and increase the risk of ingrowing hairs and hair follicle infections. Trim hair using a bikini trimmer.

▶ Saddle soreness isn't an inevitable part of cycling and, if you're suffering from it, something's not right.

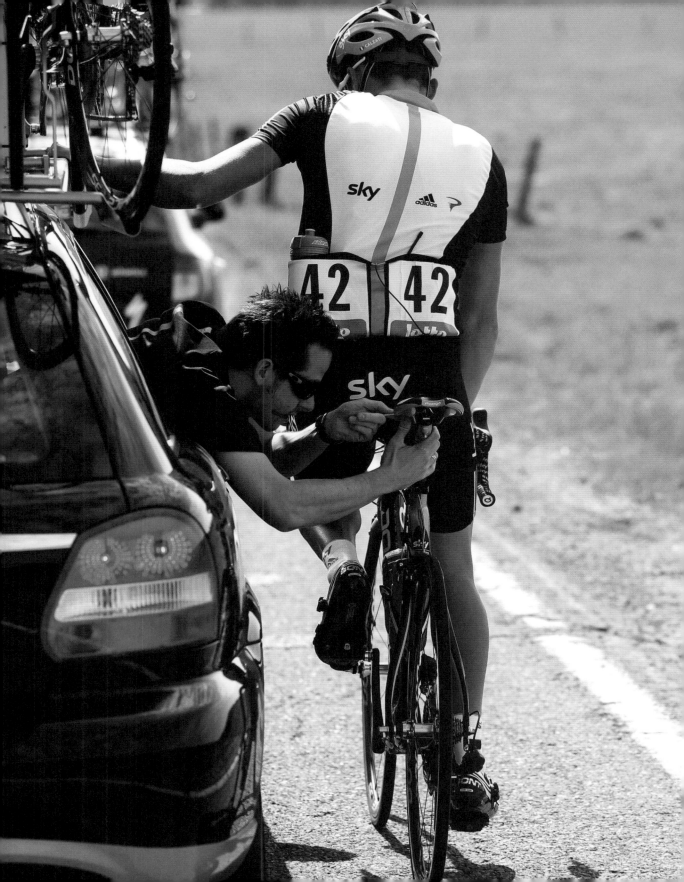

Indoor trainer

If you're serious about improving your cycling, an indoor trainer is an absolute essential. All of the midweek workouts in this book are best suited to being completed on an indoor trainer. You'll get plenty of riders who'll say 'man up and get out on the roads', but they're completely missing the point. You don't ride indoors to escape the weather, you ride indoors because it's the best way to maximise the benefits you'll get from training, especially if your time is limited. Riding indoors isn't a soft option, far from it. I'd take an outdoor ride every time, no matter what the weather, but I know that the indoor trainer is the key to becoming a better rider. You can ride at exactly the right intensity for exactly the right amount of time and focus 100 per cent on the effort you're making. There's no distraction of other road users, no junctions to slow down for and, when you're having to dig in really deep for that final push, you don't have to worry about a car pulling out in front of you or not seeing a pothole. Yes, riding indoors is boring, yes, you get uncomfortably sweaty and yes, most sessions are painful, but the gains are definitely worth it.

Turbo vs rollers vs static bike

Choosing an indoor trainer can be a fairly bewildering and overwhelming retail experience, with a huge number of makes, models and types to choose from. With both a turbo and rollers, you use your existing bike, either bolting it to the turbo or simply riding on the rollers. A static bike is a stand-alone piece of kit.

For the majority of riders, the most affordable and flexible option is probably a turbo. The newer direct-drive ones are especially good and, from a workout perspective, will cover almost all eventualities. However, I can't emphasise the bike handling and pedalling technique benefits of rollers enough. If you have the space and the budget, getting both is really the best option. Warm up, cool down and do leg speed and recovery spins workouts on the rollers, and use the turbo for the hard yards.

The main thing is to find an indoor training solution that works for you and that you will use. Indoor training isn't fun and, as you'll normally be doing it at the end of a long day at work, any excuse or obstacle, mental or physical, to overcome can easily break your resolve.

'In my professional days it [turbo trainer] would have been the first piece of equipment I would have saved from a fire. Reaching your full potential will almost be impossible without it.'

GRAEME OBREE, DOUBLE BREAKER OF THE WORLD HOUR RECORD, DOUBLE INDIVIDUAL PURSUIT WORLD CHAMPION AND CYCLING INNOVATOR

	Turbo	Rollers	Static bike
What is it?	A turbo trainer is a metal frame that you bolt your bike to using a special rear QR skewer. A roller then presses against your rear tyre and, by using a fan, fluid or magnets, generates resistance for you to pedal against. Direct drive trainers replace the roller against your rear tyre with a cassette that your drivetrain drives directly. They're generally quieter, deliver more consistent performance and don't chew up your rear tyre.	Three drums mounted in a frame that you ride on. A rubber belt connects one of the rear rollers to the front one so that your front wheel rotates too. Most makes and models are similar in design but the profile, shape, size and material of the drums does vary. Most offer limited, if any, resistance options and only top-end models will produce ride data.	A dedicated stationary bike varying from cheap and cheerful 'fitness models' from your local catalogue store to high-end commercial models.
Cost	£100 – £1,500 +	£150 – £1,500	£100 – £2,250
What to look for and what to avoid	It can be tempting to go for a cheap and cheerful turbo but it's likely to be unbearably noisy, not feel realistic and put you off using it. You can get a good workout with a mid-price turbo, especially if you already have a power meter on your bike, so don't think you have to get one that displays loads of data and metrics. Do look for variable resistance, though, and a handlebar-mounted lever to alter it with.	If you're fairly new to rollers, look for wider drums and a parabolic shape, which helps keep you in the centre. The bearings and sturdiness of some budget sets of rollers can be poor. If you're planning on using them for pre-race warm-ups or need to store them away after use, ensure they have a good folding mechanism.	Avoid low-price fitness models like the plague. The experience of riding won't be anything like riding on the road and it'll probably just end up as a clothes horse. Spinning-style bikes can be good as the fixed flywheel can aid the development of a smooth and even pedalling technique. However, training feedback is minimal or non-existent and the resistance mechanisms can be fairly crude. You really do get what you pay for with static bikes. If you definitely want one, get a Wattbike or similar.
Pros	You can find a turbo for most budgets and there are always plenty of second-hand ones. You'll probably be using your regular bike so your position will be spot on. If you're short on space, many fold top flat. You can generate plenty of resistance so they are good for high power and strength efforts.	Brilliant for developing balance, bike handling skills, smooth pedalling technique and leg speed. You can get a decent set of second-hand rollers fairly cheaply. You'll be riding your normal bike so your position will be correct. Less tyre wear than a turbo.	If you've got the space, a stationary bike is always set up and ready to go and there's no need to bring your road bike indoors. Higher end models offer an amazing amount of feedback, data and flexibility.
Cons	Non-direct drive models can chew up your rear tyre. Consider investing in a turbo-specific tyre or even a dedicated rear wheel and cassette. If you do go for a budget trainer, expect it to be noisy. As your bike is locked in place, you won't be developing your balance or bike handling skills.	With less resistance, they're not suited to higher power efforts. You may have to invest some time in learning to ride them before you can start doing proper workouts.	You will have to spend a fair amount to get a model that's worthwhile. You'll need space to leave it permanently set up. You might struggle to exactly replicate your riding position.

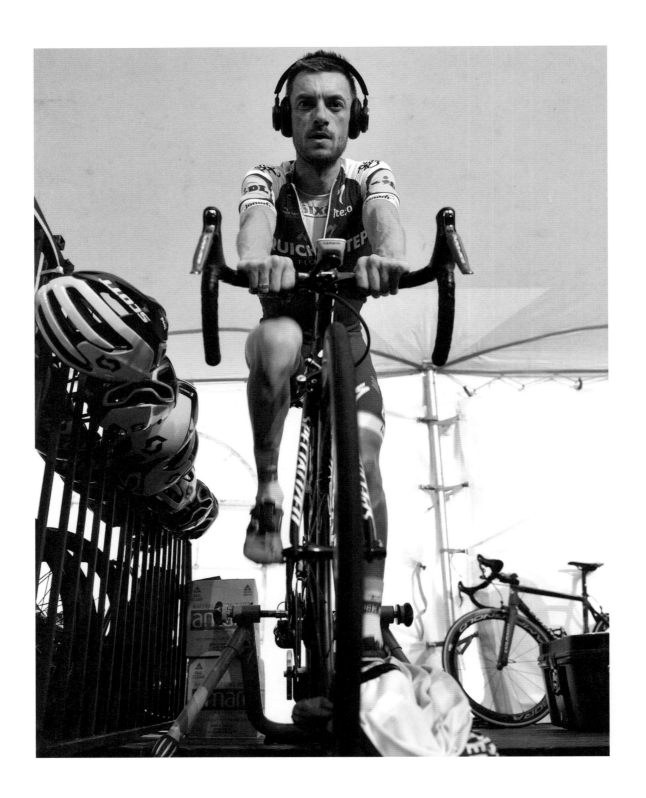

'You can get so much structure and benefit from using an indoor trainer. Pros can get out and ride during the day but, especially during the winter, if you can only ride early in the morning or in the evening, they're brilliant. For me I just never felt safe or that I was getting a quality training session when riding in the dark dodging cars and potholes. It's time efficient, you can get a really good session done in an hour.'

DEAN DOWNING, EX-PRO, FORMER BRITISH CIRCUIT RACE CHAMPION AND NOW COACH

Although professional riders will use indoor trainers, especially for pre-race warm-ups and post-race cool-downs, most won't put the hours in on them that non-pros do. The simple reason for this is that most pros will overwinter in a climate that's more amenable to riding. They're not tied by work to early mornings or evenings and will gravitate to areas that provide ideal roads and climbs for the workouts they need to do.

LEARNING TO RIDE ROLLERS

If you do decide to opt for rollers, don't get too stressed about learning to ride them, it's really not that hard. You manage to hold a straight line on the road and rollers are no different. It's also a myth that, if you do come off the rollers, you'll go shooting across the room. You may have an embarrassing little tumble but that'll be it. There are some great technique videos available on the internet and here are some key pointers to follow.

- The best place to set up your rollers when you're learning is in a doorway. This allows you to lean against the frame if you lose your balance without having to take your hands off the bars.
- Make sure you adjust the length of the rollers so that the front roller sits just in front of your front axle.
- Having to clip in can freak some riders out so, until you're confident, put on some flat pedals and trainers.
- Stay relaxed and don't grip your bars too hard. If you're tense, you'll overreact to the bike moving underneath you and make it feel twitchy.
- Don't look down at your front wheel – you wouldn't do this when you're riding on the road. Place a water bottle or track pump on the floor 1½–2 bike lengths in front of the rollers. This will give you something to focus on and help you with your balance.
- Once you get going, listen to the pitch and volume of the whir the rollers are making. If it's constantly changing, your pedal stroke is uneven. A smooth and even sound means that your pedal stroke is the same.

◄ An indoor trainer is essential to maximise your cycling potential, especially if you're pressed for time and fitting training around work and family commitments.

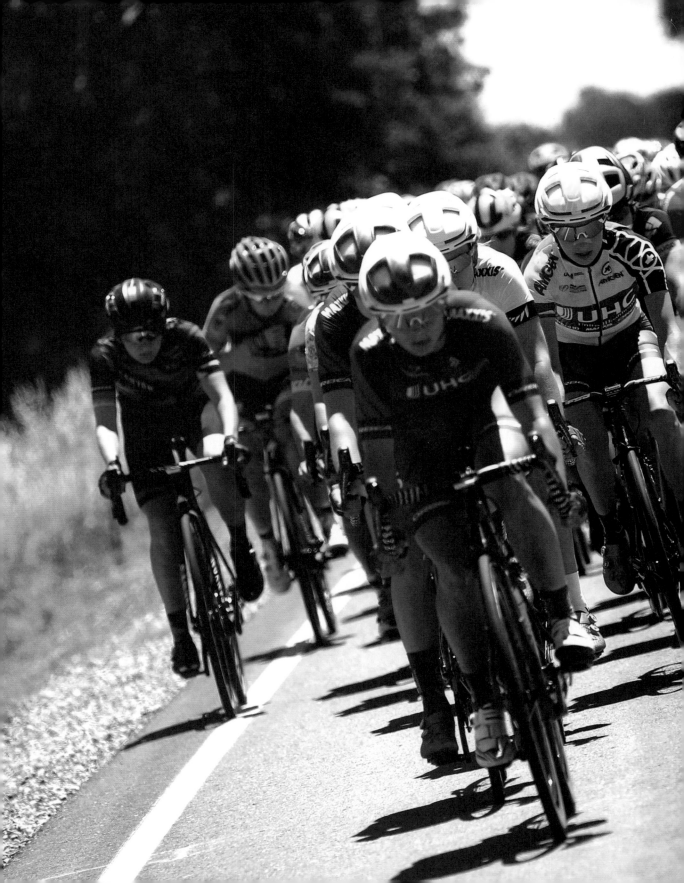

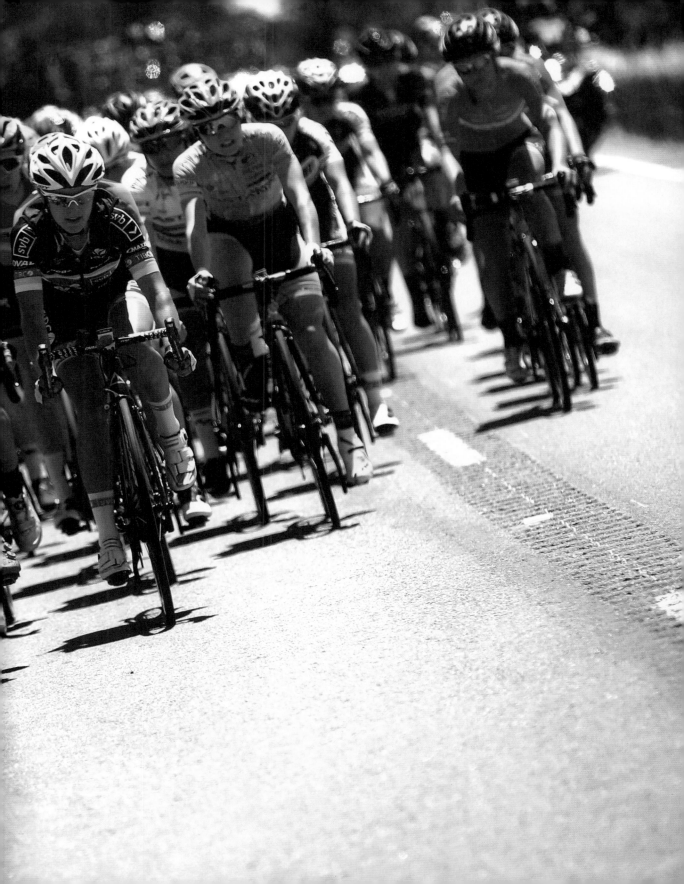

Virtual reality

Virtual reality trainers have been around for a while, but with improved smart trainers and subscription packages such as Zwift, the degree of interaction and closeness to real riding has massively improved. There's already a large community of riders who 'meet up' for group rides and even race online. The experience is becoming increasingly sophisticated, with the trainer adjusting for sitting on the wheel of another rider or even for hitting a sector of cobbles. It's a lot of fun and can certainly help to boost your motivation levels. It's important, though, to remember that an indoor trainer shouldn't become a complete substitute for riding outdoors. They're brilliant for those focused sessions that are difficult to complete outdoors or for when the weather makes riding on the road dangerous. However, whenever possible, longer endurance-style rides should be done outdoors and not on an indoor trainer. Spend too much time on an indoor trainer during the winter and you'll definitely find that your bike handling skills will have suffered when you do finally emerge into the great outdoors in the spring.

There's no doubt that the sophistication and applications of virtual reality to cycling are going to evolve rapidly. During a presentation at the International Cyclefit Symposium 2016, Dr Scott Drawer, head of Sky Performance Hub, the man charged by Team Sky to develop the next marginal gains, talked about the potential of virtual reality. He envisaged similar set-ups to Formula 1, where sophisticated simulators allow extensive testing. A rider's position or bike set-up could be altered and then, with a 100 per cent realistic simulated riding experience and performance analysis, the impact of those changes could be assessed. We've already seen Belgian company Bioracer develop a virtual wind tunnel that uses green-screen technology, and should make aero testing affordable and more widely available.

Setting up your pain cave

As we've already seen, you have to make your indoor trainer set-up as alluring as possible. You might not necessarily want to do the sessions or look forward to them, but don't make your set-up your excuse to avoid doing them.

Getting started is the hardest bit of any session, so make it as easy as possible. The ideal is to find a location where you can leave your trainer set up and ready to go. If you're using a turbo-specific tyre to save wear on your road tyres, there's no way you'll

INDOOR CYCLING CLASSES

If, for whatever reason, you can't get an indoor trainer or can't find the motivation to ride one, indoor group cycling classes can be an option. However, you need to be careful about the class you pick and ideally should look for one that's led by a cyclist. You should be able to use your own cycling shoes but might struggle to accurately replicate your riding position. You won't be able to do the exact workouts prescribed in the book and, unless you're lucky enough to belong to a gym with a fleet of Wattbikes, training feedback is likely to be limited and often completely subjective. If your gym does have Wattbikes or similar, though, and you can use them outside of class times, this can be a great option for those midweek sessions.

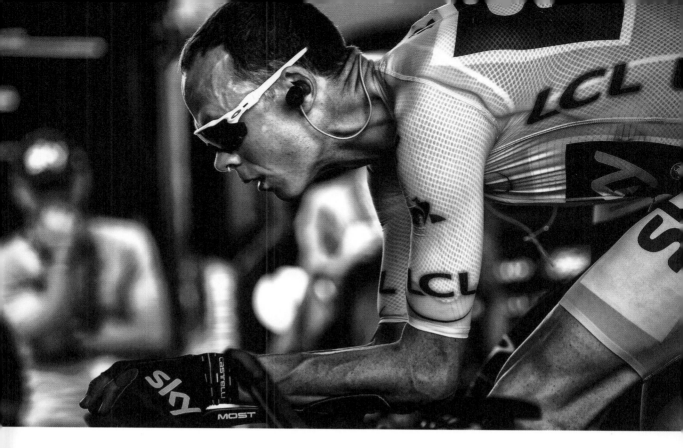

go through the faff of changing a tyre prior to a session. Buy a cheap second-hand rear wheel, a lower-tier-compatible cassette, and then you'll just need to swap a wheel in. Even that can prove too much of an obstacle, though, so if you know your next session is a turbo workout, set it up at the end of your previous one. Make sure all of your kit is laid out and ready to go, bottles filled and tyres pumped up. Have all of your devices pre-synched – tech issues can easily break your resolve.

Think carefully about where you're going to site your trainer. The shed at the bottom of the garden might seem like a good idea, but does it have a power supply and will you fancy traipsing out to it in the pouring rain? Make sure the room is cool and well ventilated and has a hard, solid floor. Garages can be perfect, but in the depths of winter you may need to wrap up until you get going. A basement or ground-floor room is the ideal as, although modern trainers are far quieter and if you site it on a rubber mat on top of some old carpet underlay, noise from vibration can be significantly reduced, flat or apartment dwellers do need to be considerate of neighbours below. Intense indoor workouts require high levels of focus and concentration so a location where you won't be distracted is preferable. Shut yourself away and make it clear that, if the trainer's whirring, you're not to be disturbed.

Even in the coolest garage, once you start riding hard on an indoor trainer, you'll start to overheat. This increases your rate of perceived exertion so if you don't attempt to keep cool, you'll be compromising the effectiveness of the workout. One, two or even three high-powered fans can make a massive difference to your comfort levels and how you perform on the indoor trainer.

You're going to sweat, so make sure you have plenty of towels and water on hand and a 'sweat thong' to protect your bike, as sweat can be really corrosive to sensitive areas such as the headset. Also, from a comfort perspective, you move less in the saddle on an indoor trainer, so decent shorts and chamois cream are musts.

If your budget doesn't stretch to a smart trainer and a virtual reality subscription, some old race footage and a decent playlist can give you a motivational boost. Wireless headphones are another worthwhile investment as a dangling cable that's a bit annoying after five minutes will drive you completely mad after an hour on the turbo.

Power meter

If you're not already objectively monitoring your riding intensity with either a heart rate monitor or a power meter and utilising training zones, you stand to make some massive gains. If this applies to you, it could be tempting to dip your toe in the water first with the cheaper option of a heart rate monitor but, although you can train reasonably well and significantly improve using a heart rate monitor, I can't urge you strongly enough to invest in a power meter. I'll confess that, having used and been fairly successful using a heart rate monitor for a number of years, I was fairly late joining the power meter party. However, when I finally succumbed in 2013, it's not hyperbole to say it revolutionised how I rode and approached my cycling training. At the time, I was racing long course duathlons, focusing on defending my age-group world title at Powerman Zofingen. Pacing the 150km (93-mile) bike leg, which was followed by

▼ Without a doubt a power meter should be top of your kit upgrade wish list. Using one will make you a better cyclist.

'I was one of the first to use a cycling computer for racing. Then in 1984 I started using a heart rate monitor to track my performance. The big one for me, though, was using watts. I was one of the first to get into power meters and that was a major transformation.'

GREG LEMOND, THREE TIME TOUR DE FRANCE WINNER AND DOUBLE WORLD CHAMPION

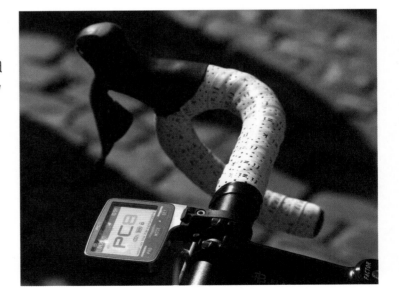

'When I first started working with professional cyclists eight or nine years ago, SRM power meters were state of the art and incredibly expensive. Now, there are more brands and they're so much more affordable. Every bike that all the riders on the team use is equipped with a power meter. Our riders would almost feel naked now without one! There's no doubt that structured training using power is the best way to improve performance. It's just a brilliant tool for maximising training efficiency.'

ANDREAS LANG, TEAM PHYSIOLOGIST, CANYON/SRAM

a hilly 30km (18½-mile) run, was crucial. Once I'd tested for my functional threshold power (FTP) and found my training zones, riding to power facilitated far more accurate and consistent pacing than I'd ever managed with a heart rate monitor. I was riding my regular training routes faster but, more importantly, feeling far fresher at the end of them. I was cutting out all of those little spikes and digs that, although barely noticeable at the time, accumulate over the course of a long ride and eventually lead to your pace tailing off. It made pacing so much easier that, especially on time trials, it almost felt like cheating. More intense intervals were no longer a guessing game, with no need to account for heart rate lag – I knew from the first pedal stroke exactly the intensity I was riding at. It also allowed me to objectively and accurately monitor my training load and to plan effective tapers and peaks. Like a bike fit, a power meter doesn't give you quite the same shiny-object-buying pleasure as a new set of fancy wheels, but it has far more potential to improve your riding.

Just for pros?

Even though the price of power meters is coming down, buying one still represents a fairly hefty financial outlay. Like saddles and bikes, you've actually got an advantage over the pros as you won't be obliged to use the power meter and head unit supplied by the team's sponsors. If you buy a power meter from one of the established manufacturers, you can be certain you're buying a professional-level product. Many riders think that their ability or the level they ride at doesn't justify buying one, but this is a mistake. I'd argue that a power meter is of more value to a time-strapped rider than to a pro. With limited time to train, optimising the training benefits of every pedal stroke is a priority and a power meter allows you to do that. It'll mean an end to junk miles and significantly reduce your risk of overtraining. Power meters are especially useful for pacing sportives and Gran Fondos. On these long and gruelling rides, often over mountainous terrain, your ability to pace well is key to riding strongly throughout the event. A power meter removes all of the guesswork from pacing. It's likely, if you're tackling an event such as L'Étape du Tour, that you'll have invested in a decent bike, put significant hours into your training and probably spent a fair bit on travel and accommodation. Getting your pacing wrong, which even the most experienced riders can do, can easily turn your big day into a disappointing hellish nightmare. Surely a device that massively minimises the risk of that happening is worth investing in? The effectiveness of power meters is demonstrated by the fact that, after the 2017 Vuelta a España, Alberto Contador called for them to be banned in races. His argument was that they allowed riders to pace their riding so well that they removed the spontaneity and aggression of racing.

Power vs heart rate

If you're still not convinced of the benefits of cycling with power, here's a summary of the pluses and minuses.

> 'I never used a power meter until I joined Canyon/SRAM. I'd never wanted one or needed one – well, I didn't think I needed one. But when I broke my ankle and I was making my recovery and comeback they just wanted to monitor my progress. I promised myself I wouldn't become a power nerd but I have!'
>
> **HANNAH BARNES**, CANYON/SRAM

- The biggest advantage of using a power meter is that the wattage you're seeing is absolute and unaffected by external variables in the way that heart rate is. Pre-event nerves, an argument with your other half before heading out for a ride or an encounter with an aggressive dog can all raise your heart rate. Conversely, illness or fatigue can depress it. Also, over the course of a long ride, a phenomenon known as cardiac drift causes your heart rate to drop relative to the effort you're putting in. You'll feel as though you're pushing hard but your heart rate will stay stubbornly low. Power is unaffected by any of these factors and gives 100 per cent accurate feedback on the output you're producing.
- There's always a lag with heart rate in responding to any change in intensity. This can present a problem for interval sessions. For example, if you're performing 5-minute Zone 5 intervals using heart rate, you'll probably find that it takes at least the first minute or so to build into the correct zone or you'll go off too hard in an attempt to get your heart rate up quickly and struggle to finish the effort. With power, you can be sure you're hitting the right intensity from the first pedal stroke and, especially for high-intensity work, this can be invaluable.
- From a training analysis and planning perspective, we're only just scratching the surface of what's possible with power meters. By using analysis software such as TrainingPeaks, power data can give you incredible insights into your training and even allow you to accurately plan tapers and peaks for key events. As more third party software developers become involved, data analysis will become increasingly sophisticated. Former Great Britain Cycling Team and Team Sky nutritionist Nigel Mitchell believes that the close relationship between pacing and fuelling is an area that will see significant advances. He's convinced that in the not-too-distant future, power meter data will be interpreted to tell you what and when to eat on the bike. We're already at the point where usable automatic gear shifting systems based on power are available and, whether you think this is

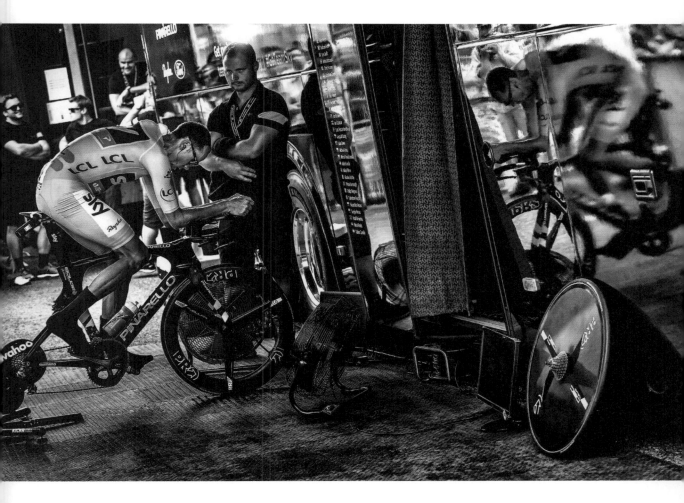

a good or a bad thing, cycling is going to become more tech- and data-heavy.

- For most riders, the main disadvantage of power is the cost, but, to reiterate, you might have to put off that wheel upgrade to get a power meter but it'll be far more beneficial to your riding. Also, as patents expire and more manufacturers enter the market, prices will continue to fall.

- Another disadvantage is that a power meter only tells you the power you're generating, it doesn't tell you how hard your body is working to produce those watts. This is why you shouldn't ditch your heart rate monitor when you get a power meter but should combine these two metrics. If you notice, for example, that, for a given power, your heart rate is elevated above what it normally would be for that output, this could be a good indicator that you might be ill or run down and need to back off a bit. Similarly, a low heart rate relative to power could indicate fatigue or that you've gained fitness and need to retest your FTP and set new training zones.

'We still use heart rate but it has its limitations. For example, if you're doing sprint training, say five to thirty second efforts, you'll always look at power first as you're wanting to see how powerful their sprint is. For longer efforts and rides, looking at heart rate is useful. If you track heart rate and power, over the course of three or four days, or three weeks on a Grand Tour, you can see how the rider's power output for a given heart rate starts to tail off as fatigue builds. If a rider normally puts out 250 watts at 160 bpm but we're only seeing 220 watts for that heart rate, this could be a sign of fatigue, overtraining or even illness.' **ANDREAS LANG**, TEAM PHYSIOLOGIST, CANYON/SRAM

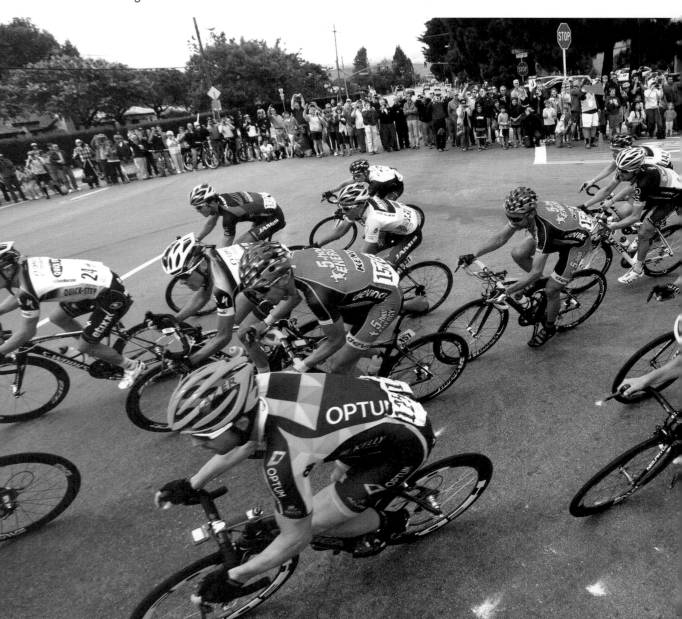

▼ In a bunch race, react to the race and not the numbers on your power meter. You can nerd out on the data afterwards.

With the glut of data that a power meter produces, it's easy to suffer from paralysis by analysis. Riders spend more time pawing over their ride data than actually riding or become robotic slaves to their power meters, losing spontaneity from their cycling. I'll sometimes tape over my power meter during a time trial, just to check that the numbers aren't limiting my performance. If I'm in a bunch race, unless I'm making a heroic solo break I won't be looking at my power meter, I'll be reacting to the riders around me. Conversely, some riders buy a power meter and never really get the most out of it. They might brag about their peak power during the café stop but, in the main, it's just an expensive and fairly redundant piece of kit on their bike. You have to invest a bit of time and effort into learning how to use one and meaningfully interpret the data but, at the same time, not become a power geek.

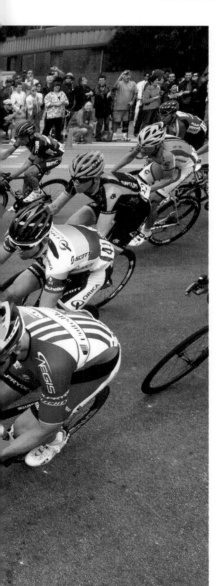

'Power meters only really became universally used towards the end of my career as a rider but now, as a coach, the more I learn about them and the data they produce, the more I realise their huge benefit. For most of the time that I was racing, it was on heart rate and feel. Years of experience meant I became pretty good at knowing when I was tired, when I'd gone hard and if I needed to back off a bit. Even with a power meter, having that self-awareness and feel is still really important. Power data won't tell you if your legs are sore or if your sit bones are aching but, if you can combine power data with good body awareness, it's brilliant. When I did start using one in my final year, it didn't make me overhaul my training but it did confirm that I trained hard and I certainly tweaked a few things and added some more structure.'

DEAN DOWNING, EX-PRO, FORMER BRITISH CIRCUIT RACE CHAMPION AND NOW COACH

Buying a power meter

When buying a power meter, it is important to avoid being tempted by some of the cheaper systems, which don't measure power directly using strain gauges but instead estimate it indirectly from speed and other metrics. The whole point of using power is that it's a more accurate way to assess your riding intensity, so why would you choose any system that's inherently inaccurate?

Although there are plenty of new manufacturers coming onto the market, it makes sense to be wary of first generation products as they tend to be plagued by glitches. There was a fascinating blog written by a clever engineering sort who took it upon himself to build his own power meter. His thought rationale was that the cost of the components, such as the key strain gauges, was low and actual assembly fairly simple, so how hard could it be? Well, he found that 95 per cent of the project was easy but getting the power meter to give data that were reliable, accurate and comparable from ride to ride was incredibly frustrating and practically impossible. It's not the components that you're paying for with a power meter, it's the R&D that have gone into nailing that final 5 per cent. If you buy a power meter from an unestablished manufacturer, they'll probably still be ironing out those 5 per cent kinks when it comes to market and you'll be an unwitting guinea pig.

One of the factors that have made power meters more affordable has been some manufacturers producing single-sided units. These measure the power from one leg and then simply double up to give a full power reading. Obviously, no human being is perfectly symmetrical and most riders have a stronger leg, but for comparing ride to ride and pacing, the inaccuracy will remain constant and is acceptable for most riders. However, if you can stretch to a two-sided system, the ability to compare sides, especially if you're rehabbing from an injury, together with the pedal stroke analysis metrics that are available, make it worthwhile. I've found that when I'm fresh and riding below FTP, my left/right balance stays at 50/50. However, when I start pushing hard or I get fatigued, my stronger right leg starts taking on the lion's share of the work.

Next, you should consider whether you'll want to swap your power meter between a number of bikes and how often you intend to do this. Rear wheel hub-based designs, as long as you're running compatible groupsets and monitor chain and cassette wear, are probably the simplest to swap back and forth as it's simply a case of changing a wheel. However, you can then be faced with the dilemma of racing on a training wheel or training through the winter on a high-end race wheel. Pedal-based systems aren't all quite as simple as changing a set of pedals, with some requiring accurate torquing, but are probably the best bet if you have multiple bikes. However, you may find you're restricted to a cleat and pedal system that doesn't suit you. If you're running the same groupset across your fleet, a non-driveside single-sided option isn't too tricky to move from bike to bike. If your power meter will be staying on one bike, driveside crank and spider-based options, such as the original SRM power meter, are reliable and accurate.

Remember that you may have to factor a head unit into your budget. If you already own a cycling computer that is ANT+ compatible, most power meters will talk to it.

There's no doubt that more options for power measurement will become available. For example, a system in the sole of cycling shoes is due on the market soon. However, before leaping on the latest technology, talk to other riders about their experiences with the various systems on the market and check out some objective reviews. I highly recommend DC Rainmaker's site for his reviews.

Additional bikes

The good news, for your bank balance at least, is that you can follow the advice in this book and become an extremely successful cyclist with just one bike. However, if you are hankering after a new bike, the following would be the best options for improving your training options and riding performance.

Winter training bike

A winter bike can double up as a commuter and will bear the brunt of wear, saving your summer bike for when speed and performance are your priorities. If you spec your winter bike with a compatible groupset to your summer bike, as you upgrade components on the latter, the cast-offs can live out their days on your winter hack. Over the course of a few winters, a dedicated winter bike can definitely recoup its cost in saved wear to your summer pride and joy. Another advantage of having a dedicated winter training bike is that you can set up your summer bike permanently for indoor training. This means no wheel- or tyre-changing hassle and no dragging a dirty bike through the house, and it makes you far less likely to bail on those gruelling indoor workouts.

I'd suggest trying to get your position as near to matching as you can on all of your bikes. Some people recommend a more relaxed position for winter but, if you've had a professional bike fit, it shouldn't be affected by the seasons. You may, however, want to choose a greater range of gears that'll allow you to spin up climbs on winter rides that specify steadier efforts.

Disc brakes make a lot of sense on a winter bike, taking the braking surface away from the mud and wet, and saving on rim wear. They also give you a bit more clearance

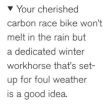
▼ Your cherished carbon race bike won't melt in the rain but a dedicated winter workhorse that's set-up for foul weather is a good idea.

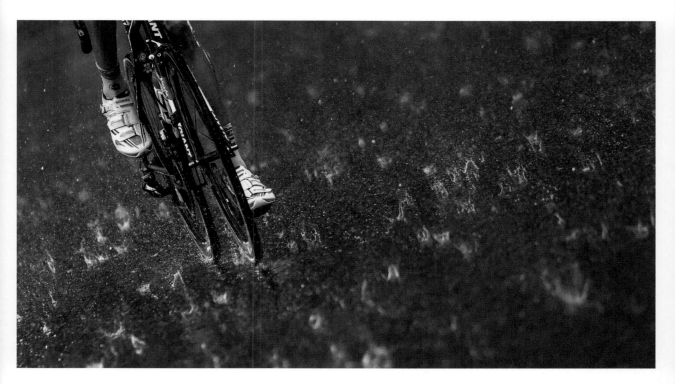

for wider tyres, giving you a bigger contact patch for improved grip and a plusher ride.

Full mudguards should be viewed as an essential for a winter bike, especially if you're joining any group rides. You can get clip-on guards for almost any bike and, although they may be a bit fiddly to fit and spoil the aesthetics slightly, they should be considered essential for winter riding. Full-length guards, with proper flaps, keep your backside and feet dry and your bike cleaner, and make yours a pleasant wheel to follow.

A slightly left field and definitely old school suggestion for a winter training bike is to go fixed. With a fixed gear, there's no freewheeling, so you earn every kilometre and you'll feel even a fairly sedate Sunday club run. You'll get high-cadence leg speed work on the flats and downhills, and big gear and low-cadence strength work on any climbs. The fixed gear also encourages you to develop a smooth and even pedal stroke, which definitely translates to regular riding. There's something quite meditative about the rhythm you settle into when riding fixed and you never have to deal with the frustration of misfiring gears. Best of all, especially if you fit full-length mudguards, cleaning and maintenance is minimal. Just run the chain through a rag, lube and occasionally tension it, and you're pretty much done. It's not for everyone, especially if you live in a very hilly area, but for a real winter workhorse fixed is definitely worth considering.

Mountain bike/cyclo-cross bike

It's no coincidence that one of the best bike handlers in the pro peloton, Peter Sagan, comes from a mountain biking background. These skills, along with providing some great photo opportunities, are one of the main reasons for his success on the road. By being so comfortable and relaxed on the bike, he saves an incredible amount of energy, which gives him a real edge when the race heats up.

Almost all road cyclists can benefit from including some off-road riding in their

▼ Riding off-road will make you a better road rider and give you a fun training option.

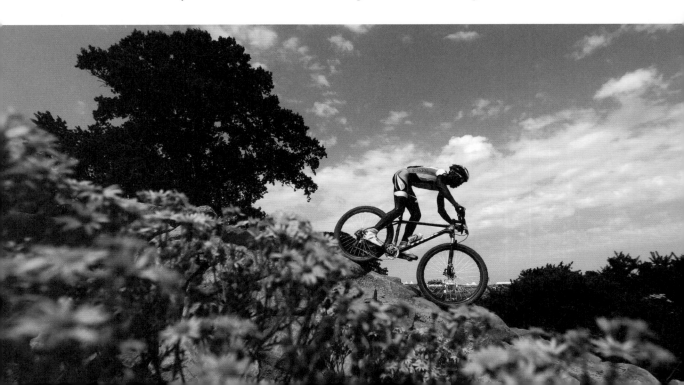

training and a mountain bike or cyclo-cross bike opens up this possibility to you. Hours spent road riding can result in a very static riding style and poor bike handling skills. Off-road cycling forces you to constantly change your riding position, learn cornering and braking skills and become an all-round better bike rider. This translates into faster all-round riding, especially on more technical roads, and a greater ability to deal with unexpected hazards such as falling riders or potholes. Icy, wet and dark winter conditions can make roads unpleasant and dangerous places to be, and being able to get off the roads gives you a safe and enjoyable winter option. Off-road cycling gives a much more interval-style workout than road cycling. This gives you a great top-end hit, and sudden steep climbs or slogs through mud are an alternative to gym sessions for building cycling-specific strength and power. Off-road cycling provides a far more total body workout than road cycling. You'll be using your upper body to soak up lumps and bumps, lift your front wheel over trail obstacles and gain extra power on steep climbs. Having to constantly shift your weight and centre of gravity to maintain traction and balance will challenge your trunk muscles in a way you'll never experience on the road. Riding off-road punishes choppy and heavy-footed pedal mashing. Try to muscle up a loose or slippery climb and you'll soon spin out and be off your bike and walking. To maintain traction, you have to develop an even, circular and smooth pedalling style. You can then transfer this pedalling technique to your road cycling where it'll result in far smoother, more economical and faster riding.

If you opt for a cyclo-cross bike, this is an incredibly versatile choice. Run it with road tyres and you've got a brilliant winter training bike. Leave the knobbly tyres on and you can explore bridleways and byways that you'd never venture on with a road bike. There is an increasing number of cyclo-cross friendly sportive-style rides, which are great fun and can add real variety and a challenge to your event schedule. Racing cyclo-cross through the winter is brilliant for bike handling skills and fitness. It's an incredibly accessible form of racing that will be covered more thoroughly in Chapter 8. It's no coincidence that, no matter what their preferred discipline, young riders working through the Great Britain Cycling Team Performance Pathway are encouraged to race cyclo-cross. For developing bike handling skills and overall fitness, it's hard to beat. With a background in cyclo-cross, Tom Pidcock, in 2017, won junior world titles in both that discipline and the time trial, and is being tipped for a great future on the road. Again, like Peter Sagan and his mountain biking background, the skills Tom has learned riding cyclo-cross make him a more relaxed and energy-efficient rider whether on- or off-road.

Adventure/gravel bike

A final option to consider, which can potentially serve all three options of winter trainer, mountain bike and crosser, is an adventure/gravel bike. These tend to have slightly less racy geometry than an all-out racing cyclo-cross bike and will also usually have drillings for mudguards and pannier racks. Some also allow you to run 650b (27½in) wheels with fatter tyres for more mountain biking type trails and then swap in 700c (29in) wheels with narrower cyclo-cross or even road tyres.

GEARING

Not so long ago, the standard gearing set-up on a road bike was 53/39t chainrings on the front and a cassette giving a range of 11–23t or 11–25t at the rear. If you wanted lower gears, you'd be looking at a triple chainset but they tended to be the preserve of tourers and recreational riders. Hills tended to be a knee-popping grind or an out of the saddle wrestling match with your handlebars. Now, though, with 11-speed cassettes giving huge 11–32t ranges and compact (50/34t) and pro or semi-compact (52/36t) chainsets, spinning higher cadences even up the steepest climbs is possible and triples have been pretty much consigned to the dusty spare parts box at your local bike shop. Mountain bikers are already using 12-speed cassettes with 10–50t ranges and road riders are modifying these set-ups for use on the road. So what gearing should you opt for and how low should you go?

Think about your fitness level and the type of riding you'll mainly be doing. For the vast majority of sportive riders, a compact (50/34t) chainset paired with an 11/12–28t cassette should cover most eventualities. If you're tackling a very hilly event or heading for some big mountains, though, you might want to consider upping the cassette to a 32t. Don't be put off by disparaging comments from old school or 'macho' riders, there's nothing tough about grinding up hills. On recent Grand Tours Chris Froome, Alberto Contador and other top contenders have been spotted running compacts and 32t cassettes. It not only allows them to maintain a more efficient seated position on steep climbs but, with the stages ahead to consider, results in less muscular stress. Also, don't worry about 'spinning out' on flats or descents. Turning your top gear of 50/11 at 100 rpm will see you travelling at just under 59kph (37mph) and, although you may go faster on long downhills, you're likely to be freewheeling. As mentioned, road riders are experimenting with even wider ranging mountain biking cassettes but, in my opinion, you can go too low with your gearing. You'll struggle to keep your front wheel down, will barely be travelling above walking pace and will have significant jumps as you shift through your gears, which can make maintaining rhythm difficult. Apart from extreme cases or specific needs, such as an injury, there should be no need to go lower than a 34t chainring paired with a 32t sprocket for road riding.

Stronger riders and those looking to race, who might want a bigger top gear, or, if you tend to favour flatter riding, a pro or semi-compact (52/36t) chainset offers a great option. You might also want to consider, if the course is suitable, running a smaller ranging cassette, such as 11–25t, as there will be less of a jump between gears. This is the set-up I have on my summer road bike that I'll ride sportives and circuit race on. For hilly routes, though, I'll change down to an 11–28t cassette.

Traditionalists, or those who ride and race predominately on the flat, may want to opt for a 53/39t chainset but, for a relatively small gain in your highest gear with the extra tooth upfront, you're likely to be sacrificing a fair amount of climbing efficiency. That said, not all of us are spinners, and a higher-gear and low-cadence approach may suit some riders better. Much has been made over recent years about the efficiency and effectiveness of high-cadence pedalling, and it certainly works for Chris Froome, but a number of studies have shown that optimal cadence is very much an individual thing. Don't become obsessed about spinning or having to maintain 90 rpm+; find the cadence that works best for you and choose the appropriate gearing that allows you to maintain it.

Other kit, clothing and equipment gains

If you've ticked all the boxes described in this chapter and are still looking for ways to buy some speed, there are certainly some seconds to be found.

As the rider accounts for 80–90 per cent of drag created, the biggest kit and equipment gains are to be made by focusing on your clothing and, as previously mentioned, your position on the bike.

Starting from the head down, aero road helmets are a fairly recent phenomenon in the pro peloton and their origins can be traced back to Mark Cavendish's win at the World Championships in 2011 when, as part of British Cycling's marginal gains philosophy, his helmet's vents were taped over to reduce turbulence and drag. The first commercially available versions weren't especially aesthetically pleasing and were met with a fair amount of derision. However, a combination of positive wind tunnel results and wins on the road have now made them the norm, especially on flat sprint stages. Gains are relatively small, typically in the 15–20 seconds range over 40km (25 miles), for an aero road helmet versus its vented equivalent. It should be noted that all 'aero gains' stats should be taken with a pinch of salt, especially if released by equipment manufacturers. The ranges given in this chapter were obtained from a number of sources and are only given as a comparative exercise. However, rider position can significantly affect this, and the gains can easily be offset by losses due to overheating

▼ With the rider accounting for the vast majority of drag, if you're putting on a rain jacket, do that zip up!

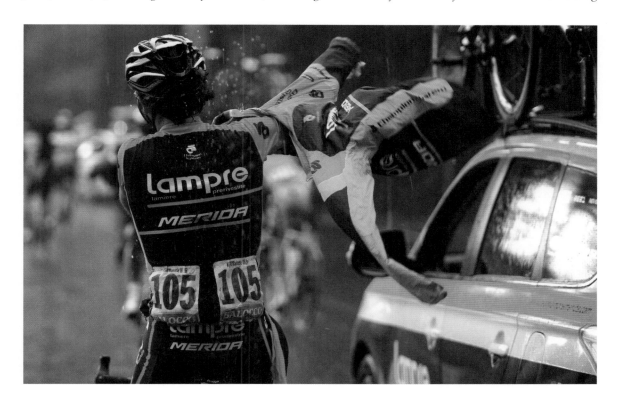

in hot conditions. For time trialists, even more outlandish aero helmet designs have become increasingly popular and, offering gains of up to a minute over 40km, can offer significant bang for your buck gains. Again though, before you rush out and buy the most aero-looking teardrop helmet you can find, this figure is an optimal best case scenario. If you tend to move your head, look down or your riding position means that the helmet's tail doesn't transition smoothly to your upper back, those gains can easily turn into losses.

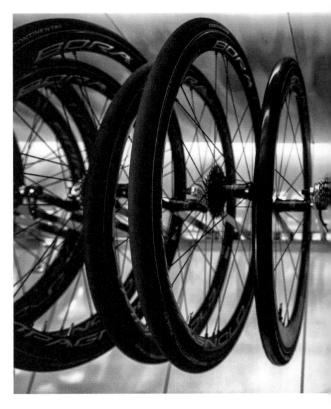

Clothing wise, if every second counts, a well-fitted high-tech skinsuit can save over 2 minutes over 40km compared with standard jersey and shorts. Again, this wasn't lost on the Great Britain Cycling Team at the 2011 World Championships, where they pioneered skinsuits for bunch races on the road. Like aero road helmets, they're now commonplace and, unlike skinsuits for track and time trials, are available with pockets for carrying spares and food. A quality skinsuit doesn't come cheap but, compared with aero upgrades to your bike, represents good value for money. If you have gone to the trouble and expense of getting a skinsuit, don't negate all the gains by pinning on your number badly. Keep it low, use plenty of pins and even look into number pockets, which can be retro fitted. For day-to-day riding and sportives, a skinsuit is probably overkill, but try to keep the aerodynamics of your clothing in mind. Fitted is always better as any audible flapping in the wind is lost speed. Do up your jersey on descents and flats, and avoid loosely fitting shell layers in poor conditions. Modern weatherproof technical jerseys allow you to stay warm, fairly dry and still aero. Another cheap but significant clothing gain, up to 30 seconds over 40km, are aero overshoes.

Also worth mentioning, while talking about the rider, are shaved legs. Specialized went to the trouble of aero testing shaved versus unshaved legs in the wind tunnel and found, for an averagely hairy rider, impressive savings of a minute over 40km. Well worth the cost of a razor! Thankfully they found much smaller gains for shaved forearms and, good news if you wear a beard, virtually none for facial hair.

If you're trying to justify buying that new aero bike, compared with sorting out your position and clothing, the cost per second saved won't help you. Like for like in terms of geometry, aero versus regular tubing will probably only save you 20–30 seconds over 40km. Similarly, the gains from aero handlebars, seat posts and such like will be fairly minimal. If all optimised they can add up, but there's definitely more significant and less costly gains to be made.

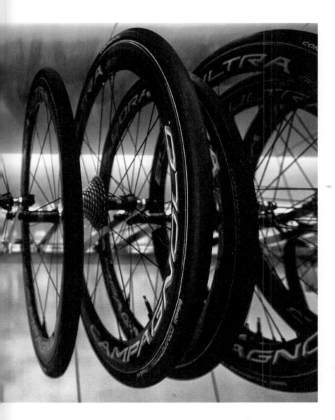

▲ Manufacturers tend to under spec wheels so, if you're looking to spend some money on your bike, your rolling stock is a good bet.

If you've bought a bike off the peg, even a fairly high-end model, upgrading the wheelset could be worthwhile. Manufacturers look to cut costs somewhere on a bike and the most common candidate is the wheels. For racing against the clock, on all but the hilliest courses a deep section or 3/5 spoke on the front and a rear disc will be the fastest, gaining 1–2 minutes over standard section wheels depending on wind conditions. For bunch events and sportives, upgrading your stock wheels to some aero and lightweight 30–50mm (1⅕–2in) wheels is definitely worthwhile. Over the course of a 5–6-hour Gran Fondo, you'll be looking at significant savings in both minutes and energy. Don't ditch your stock wheels, though – keep them for training and winter duties. With a greater understanding of aerodynamics, an area that has received a lot of attention recently has been the relationship between the tyre and the rim. This can be crucial, and it's easy to totally negate the aero benefits of your wheels by running the wrong tyre. The current trend for wider rims and wider tyres gives a smooth aero transition from rim to tyre and consistently tests faster in the wind tunnel. Most wheel manufacturers now make tyre recommendations to use with their products. Additionally, this wider rim and tyre set-up facilitates lower tyre pressures which, contrary to the previously held 'narrow and hard is faster' wisdom, reduces rolling resistance and increases speed. Taking the time to experiment with tyre pressure and adjusting it to the conditions can make a significant difference to how your bike performs. Exact set-up depends massively on rider weight and preferences but, once you've found what works best for you, checking tyre pressure should always be part of your pre-ride check. A final note on tyres is that although lightweight high performance tyres can feel great, the time they could save you over a long event has to be weighed up against the time it'll take you to fix a flat. The pros are lucky enough to have a following car with spare wheels; we're not so fortunate, so running more robust and resilient tyres is probably the wise choice.

When it comes to measurable performance boosts, upgrading your groupset probably represents one of the poorest returns for money spent. You might save a couple of hundred grams by speccing top-tier components but the difference in performance to mid-tier is negligible. Electronic shifting is trickling down to mid-tier groupsets now and, although it's probably not going to save you measurable time, its slickness and reliability, assuming you remember to charge it, is impressive.

Disc brakes have revolutionised mountain biking and cyclo-cross and, as of November 2017, have been made legal in bunch road races in the UK, Australia and

America at all levels of the sport. With the main limiting factor to braking performance being the tyres' contact patch with the road, the benefit to actual stopping distance is debatable. However, for sportives and Gran Fondos, especially on mountainous routes, they're definitely worth considering if you're buying a new bike. On long descents, there's no risk of rims overheating and potential tyre blowouts. Additionally, for winter riding especially, disc brakes mean that your rims are no longer effectively very expensive sacrificial components.

Whatever bike you ride or components you spec on it, getting into a good maintenance routine offers marginal gains and minimises maximal losses. A well-maintained bike is less likely to suffer from ride-ending mechanical failure and, for consistent training, you have to be able to rely on your bike day in and day out. Basic cleaning and drivetrain maintenance is a bare minimum, and a clean and well-lubed chain can easily save you a not insignificant 10 watts. Chain lubricant technology is a really hot topic at the moment, with secret wax, molybdenum and Teflon blends closely guarded secrets. It was rumoured that the cost of preparing Bradley Wiggins's chain for his hour record in 2015 was upwards of £6,000. There's probably no need to go this far, but keeping your chain clean and maybe even considering a waxed chain for key events will make you faster. Poorly indexed gears cause frustration, wasted energy and, as was the case with Andy Schleck and Alberto Contador in 2010, a dropped chain was a Tour-determining event. Like flapping clothing, any excessive drivetrain noise is wasted energy. Check your tyres after each ride for embedded flints or glass, as that can be a puncture waiting to happen on your next ride, potentially your big event for the year. You don't need to become a pro bike mechanic, but by developing a basic understanding of how your bike works and how to maintain it, you can improve your performance.

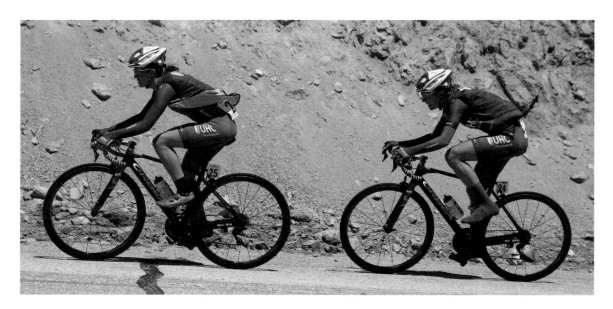

How to improve your cycling performance

▼ We all like carbon bling but there are plenty of ways to get faster without spending loads of cash.

Spend your money wisely

You can improve massively as a rider without spending a lot of money. However, if you are looking to invest some money in your riding, don't be seduced by bling upgrades.

Professional bike fit

If your bike isn't correctly fitted, you'll never achieve your true cycling potential. A quality bike fit should be a priority for all riders. Ideally, look for a physiotherapist-led bike fit using a modern motion capture system.

Indoor trainer

Not a soft option for avoiding bad weather but a vital tool for focused training. Invest time in considering the type of indoor trainer that best suits your needs and in setting it up so that you'll want to use it.

Power meter

A genuine game changer that's definitely worth the investment. Prices will continue to drop and, if you're looking for one upgrade that has the potential to transform your riding, this is it.

Second or third bike

Far from essential but can definitely facilitate training and add variety to your riding. Road cyclists have massive amounts to gain, in both fitness and bike handling skills, from hitting the trails on a mountain bike or cyclo-cross bike.

Maintenance

A clean bike is a fast bike. Any drivetrain noise or creaking or rubbing elsewhere on the bike means wasted watts that can easily cancel out the gains of aero wheels or frameset. Also, you need to have 100% confidence in your bike, especially when descending, so knowing it's well maintained is a must.

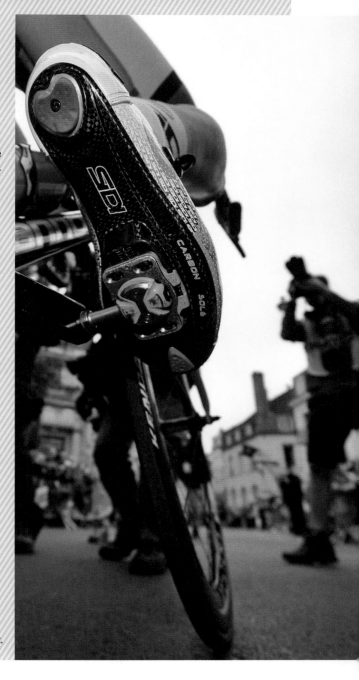

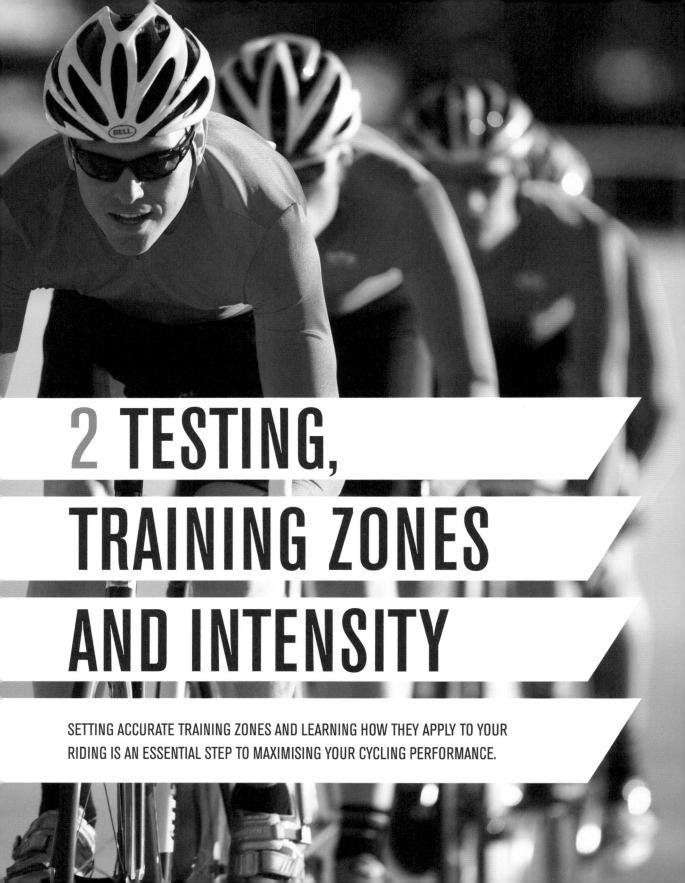

2 TESTING, TRAINING ZONES AND INTENSITY

SETTING ACCURATE TRAINING ZONES AND LEARNING HOW THEY APPLY TO YOUR RIDING IS AN ESSENTIAL STEP TO MAXIMISING YOUR CYCLING PERFORMANCE.

'It never gets easier, you just go faster.' **GREG LEMOND**

WHETHER YOU'RE TRAINING, riding a sportive or racing, it is essential to have an awareness of how hard you're working and the effect of this work on your body. Accurate pacing and being able to judge intensity are probably the key determinants of cycling success. If you don't have a way to objectively measure intensity, you're riding blind and almost guaranteed not to reach your true potential. How quickly you burn through your body's carbohydrate stores, whether you can tap into fat reserves, whether you can take on and process more fuel, and how long your leg muscles can keep working are all determined by the intensity at which you're riding. The majority of problems that riders typically encounter, including cramping, digestive distress or simply running out of gas, can usually be accounted for by poor pacing and intensity awareness. If you try to ride on feel alone, you're likely to struggle. An intensity that may feel okay on the first climb of a ride, when you're fresh and buoyed up by the excitement of the day, is likely to be above your ability and you'll end up paying for it later on. From a training perspective, unless you're able to monitor accurately the intensity you're riding at, you won't be able to ensure that you're targeting the correct physiological system that the specific session demands. Most riders who fail to monitor their riding intensity end up riding too slowly when they should be going hard and too fast when they should be taking it easy. They tend to settle into the same intensity for every ride, which fails to stimulate their bodies to adapt and become fitter, and just accumulates fatigue. It's a 'physiological no-man's-land' that inevitably results in diminishing returns, training plateaus and frustration.

> 'When I'm training, for the majority of my workouts, I train alone and it's all about hitting the numbers. Easy rides will tend to be social but, when I do these rides with friends who aren't pros, they're always staggered just how slow I go. I always tell them, I promise you, you will want to go harder than I go. It's hard to find someone who can train with me when I'm going hard but it's harder to find someone who can ride easy with me and not just drop me.'
> **PHIL GAIMON**, EX-PRO WITH GARMIN-SHARP AND CANNONDALE DRAPAC

Setting and using training zones

If you're unfamiliar with training using either a heart rate monitor or a power meter, the information in this chapter might appear initially to be a bit daunting, slightly intimidating and complicated. However, stick with it and, once you start applying it to your own riding, it'll soon start making sense. Even if you don't feel that you're quite ready to embark on a full structured training plan or are only just starting to develop your cycling fitness, investing and starting to use a heart rate monitor is still a good idea. You can begin to learn how your heart rate correlates to your perceived effort, what heart rate you can sustain on climbs and when you're pushing into the

◀ Without an objective and personalised measure of how hard you're riding, you're effectively riding blind.

red. In doing this and beginning to develop an idea of riding intensity and increased body awareness, when you do decide to take the next step and follow the testing and zone setting methods described in this chapter, it'll be far more intuitive.

What we're looking to do, by using a simple test, is find either the heart rate or power output that you're able theoretically to sustain for an hour. This level is known as functional threshold (FT). If using power, it's referred to as functional threshold Power (FTP) and if using heart rate, functional threshold heart rate (FTHR). It's an incredibly relevant metric to endurance performance as it's effectively your 'red-line intensity'. Ride below it and you'll be able to sustain the effort, go above it and you're on limited time. Once you know this key value, you can then use it to calculate accurate and personalised training zones. These zones, which are described in detail later in the chapter, range from Zones 1 and 2, representing steady paced endurance riding, through Zone 4, which encompasses that key FT value, and right to the near maximal efforts of Zone 6. Because you've tested for your FTP or FTHR, these zones will accurately reflect your personal cycling ability and physiology at that moment in time. By using them to pace your cycling, you'll be able to ensure that you're riding conservatively enough on endurance rides to last the distance and pushing hard enough on intense interval sessions to stimulate physiological change in your body. Trying to train without using accurate training zones would be analogous to attempting to drive without a speedometer, rev counter or fuel gauge.

▼ Knowing your Functional Threshold is the key to accurate pacing on the bike.

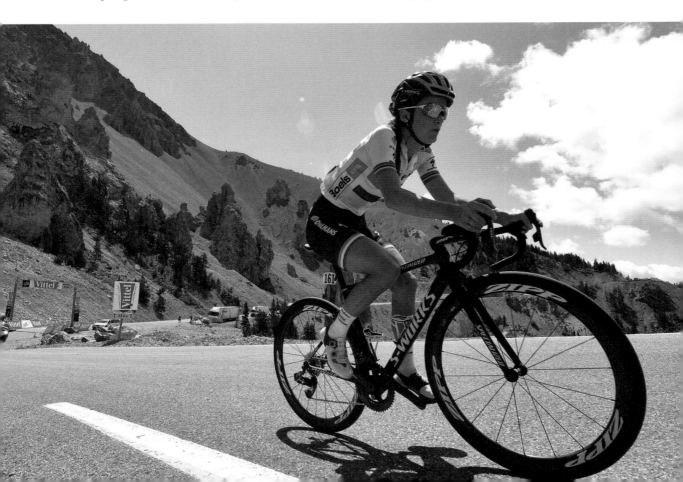

FTP vs FTHR

As discussed in Chapter 1, there are a number of considerable advantages to training with a power meter and you should make buying one your number one upgrade priority. Their use has become ubiquitous among pro cyclists, and although they have their critics, who say they reduce the spontaneity and excitement of racing, that's only because they're such effective pacing tools. The testing protocol for FTP and FTHR is the same and if you have a power meter and a heart rate monitor, you can find both figures during the same test. However, for the reasons previously discussed, you should base your training zones around FTP and train predominately using power. It's valuable, though, to have an awareness of your FTHR and heart rate zones, as major discrepancies between the two sets of zones can be an indicator that something is amiss. For example, if you were riding in Zone 2 according to power but your heart rate put you in Zone 4, this could be indicative of illness or excessive fatigue. If buying a power meter is completely out of the question, you can still train well and achieve great results using heart rate alone. However, get saving and put off buying those new wheels, I promise it's worthwhile.

Functional threshold over maximum heart rate

There are many training plans and coaches that advocate the use of maximal heart rate to set training zones. However, this is largely a training relic and the use of FT, whether heart rate or power, is now ubiquitous across the sport. British Cycling trialled it with all levels of riders, from the Great Britain Cycling Team to novice sportive riders, and found it to be the most practical and accurate way to easily calculate training zones.

There are a number of problems with using maximal heart rate. Pushing yourself to your genuine maximal heart rate is very painful, and both physiologically and psychologically extremely difficult. In fact, there are credible theories that suggest that going to your true maximum might actually be impossible, with your body effectively having its own safety cut-off. You need to be incredibly motivated to push that hard and, if you are not quite up for it, your result will be significantly off. If you're not properly rested or have an underlying bug or virus, which may not even manifest any symptoms, you won't be able to get anywhere near to your maximum. However, the sub-maximal effort of an FT test is less affected and is therefore a far more robust test.

Also, unless you're a track sprinter, your maximal heart rate isn't especially relevant to your performance. However, the intensity that you're able to sustain for an extended period is pertinent to practically all other areas of cycling performance. It therefore makes sense to test for this value and to base subsequent training zones on it.

Using generic age-based formulae

An apparently simple way to find a theoretical maximum heart rate and set training zones is to use a generic age-based formula. The classic one is deducting your age from 220 to determine a maximal heart rate figure. However, the original studies that came up with this formula never intended it to be used for performance focused training. They were looking at a safe and conservative method for estimating activity intensity for cardiac rehabilitation patients. Variations on this formula, such as the Karvonen formula, which also factors in resting heart rate, are no better really than the original as they still rely on clumping athletes together by the sweeping generalisation of age. The maximal heart rate figure that such formulas yield tends to be wildly inaccurate and therefore any zones calculated from it will be too.

Although simply plugging your age into a formula is a lot easier than performing an FTHR test from a personal effort point of view, there's no comparison between the two resulting sets of training zones. One set is personalised, accurate and tuned to your current fitness level, whereas the other is little better than a random guess. Incidentally, many of the training zone auto calculate functions on heart rate monitors use a variation of these formulae. They should be overridden and custom zones based on FTHR entered instead.

How to test

As already stated, FT is the intensity that you should be able to sustain for an hour, so it makes sense that the way to test it is to go out, ride an hour-long time trial and record your average heart rate and power for the effort. Realistically, however, it takes a huge amount of motivation, mental strength and pacing experience to ride such a time trial, and finding a suitable route for such an effort is very difficult. Fortunately, it's been shown that a 20–30-minute test can be used to deduce FT accurately, and the results I've taken from such tests do correlate very strongly to approximately hour-long race efforts such as a 40km (25 mile) time trial. Even shorter protocols are available, 8 minutes being popular, but these have been known to give inflated results.

There are a number of different protocols available for a 20–30-minute test, but the aspect common to all of them is a 20-minute effort where you go as hard as you can and record your average heart rate or power. Where they tend to differ is the warm-up and efforts prior to the recorded 20-minute one. My personal preference is the British Cycling protocol, described below, but if you find another method that you prefer, that's fine as long as you use it consistently.

The key requirements for the test are:

1   That you are well rested, having had at least one full recovery day before performing the test.
2   That you avoid eating for 2–3 hours before the test. This will vary from rider

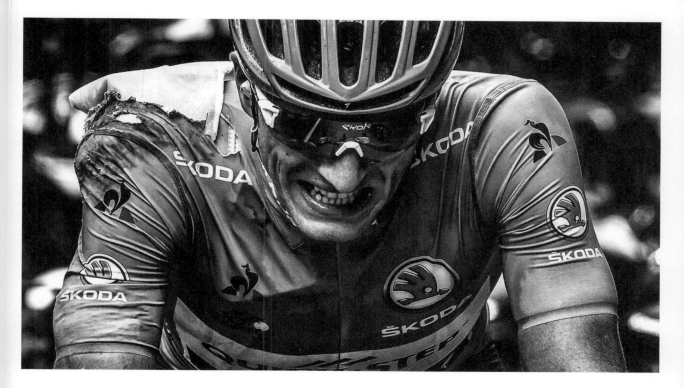

▲ Testing for
Functional Threshold
isn't pleasant but it's
definitely worthwhile.

to rider but you should follow the same nutritional protocol that you would before an intense training session. If you're unsure about this, you can find guidelines in Chapter 6.

3   If performing the test outdoors, that you have a route that allows you to ride continuously for 30 minutes without significant downhill stretches or having to stop for junctions.

4   If performing the test indoors, that you're able to record and replicate the settings on your bike and indoor trainer.

5   A heart rate monitor and/or power meter that allows you to record and recall your average heart rate or power for the test period.

FT test protocol

Warm up for at least 20 minutes. Once you know your FT and training zones, you can use the session warm-up described in Chapter 4, but if it's your first time performing the test, raise the intensity gradually so you feel as though you're working fairly hard 15 minutes in. Spin easily for the final 5 minutes.

Ride as hard as you can sustain for 30 minutes. Aim to hold a consistent cadence. On a flat course this should be in the 90–100 rpm range but may be lower if testing on a climb.

Ten minutes in, hit the lap button to record your average heart and/or power for the final 20 minutes of the effort.

Note this figure and then cool down with at least 10 minutes of easy spinning.

'Sometimes we'll test the riders' FTP in a laboratory but we'll usually test out on the road, often on a climb in Majorca. Over the last 5–6 years working with professional riders I've seen how test data correlates to training zones and whether riders are able to ride and train in those zones. Field testing definitely yields far more usable zones than testing in a laboratory. It's a real life effort and so produces real life zones that the riders can genuinely relate to and ride to. Typical laboratory protocols on an ergometer will ramp up the power every 2 minutes or so and then determine FTP from these values. However, FTP is a sustained output, up to an hour, so it's no wonder that the zones produced from laboratory tests can be unrealistic. On a real climb you can be sure that the numbers they produce are a value that they can sustain.

For testing, we'll typically use climbs that take 15–30 minutes to ride. The riders will warm up for 30–45 minutes by riding to the climb and then we'll ask them to go up the climb hard. They'll know how long the climb is and we'll make sure that they ride a consistent effort, not going off too hard. If they're motivated and well rested, they'll ride at FTP.' **ANDREAS LANG**, TEAM PHYSIOLOGIST, CANYON/SRAM

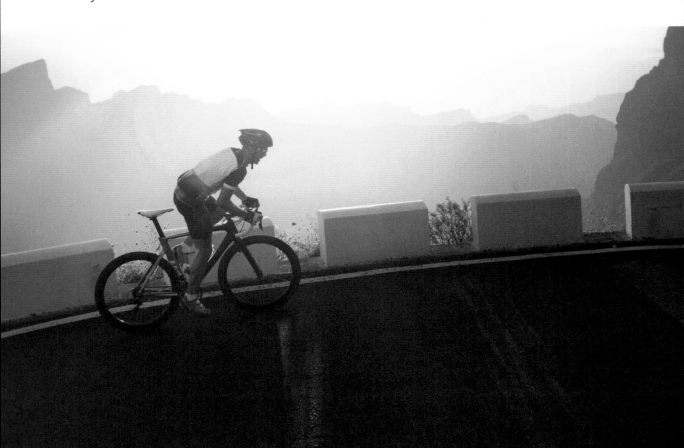

Setting zones

If training using heart rate, the average heart rate you achieved during the 20-minute effort equates to your FTHR.

If training using power, you need to subtract 5 per cent from the average power achieved during the 20-minute effort to find your FTP.

Example: Average power from 20-minute test = 250 watts. FTP = 250 × 0.95 = 237 watts

You can then calculate your training zones by applying the percentage bands in the tables below to your FTHR or FTP respectively.

HEART RATE TRAINING ZONES

Zone	Low end (% of FTHR)	High end (% of FTHR)
1	n/a	67%
2	68%	82%
3	83%	93%
4	94%	105%
5	106%	120%
6	n/a	n/a

POWER TRAINING ZONES

Zone	Low end (% of FTP)	High end (% of FTP)
1	n/a	55%
2	56%	75%
3	76%	90%
4	91%	105%
5	106%	120%
6	121	150

Once you have these zones, you'll be able to apply them to all of your riding. Program them into your bike computer, heart rate monitor or power meter head unit, or, if you're a bit old school like me, print them out and tape them to your stem.

You'll notice that no percentage band is given for heart rate Zone 6. This is because, at this high intensity, any effort would be over by the time you'd elevated your heart rate to the designated level. Many riders also struggle to pace Zone 5 for this reason and this perfectly illustrates one of the benefits of training with power. Right from the first couple of pedal strokes, you know you're in the correct zone.

Understanding training zones

Now you have your training zones, it's important to understand what they mean and how they apply to your riding.

ZONE 1: ACTIVE RECOVERY

What it feels like: Very easy. In this zone, your perceived effort shouldn't be much above brisk walking. You should be easily able to maintain a full conversation and experience no sensations of fatigue.

When you'd be in this zone: Recovery workouts, sitting in the wheels on a club run on the flat or freewheeling downhill. You'll also 'spin easy' in Zone 1 during warm-ups, cool-downs and rest periods during interval sessions.

◀ Laboratory based testing is great for research but, as you'll be riding on the road, you should test on it too.

ZONE 2: ENDURANCE

What it feels like: This should still feel sustainable and comfortable, and you should still be able to maintain a conversation fairly easily. However, especially towards the upper end of the zone or after a long time spent in it, you may have to start concentrating to maintain it.

When you'd be in this zone: Also known as 'extensive endurance', this is the go-to intensity for the bulk of a long sportive or endurance ride.

ZONE 3: TEMPO

What it feels like: Sometimes referred to as 'intensive endurance', this is a sustainable but purposeful effort. You have to concentrate to hold this intensity, any conversation would be in shorter sentences and, after time spent in this zone, you'll start to experience sensations of fatigue.

When you'd be in this zone: Longer 'tempo efforts' typically of 20–40 minutes duration. During a sportive, you would be pushing up into this zone on sustained climbs.

ZONE 4: THRESHOLD

What it feels like: The upper end of this zone is what you sustained during your FT test, so you know what it feels like. Hard sustainable discomfort is a good description, with any conversation limited to short one-word answers. This is your red-line zone and you're hovering right on the edge of what you can sustain. Expect burning legs and hard breathing.

When you'd be in this zone: In theory, FT is sustainable for an hour but you'd have to be extremely motivated and well trained. Time trialists will target this intensity for a 40km (25 mile) event. However, in training, threshold efforts are normally in the 15–20-minute range. For tough climbs on long rides, you may well go into this zone, but remember, this is your red line and holding it for too long may come back to bite you later on.

ZONE 5: VO2

This is the intensity where you're working at your absolute aerobic limit, breathing in and using the maximal amount of oxygen you can. In a sports performance lab, this point can be tested to give a value of millilitres of oxygen per kilogram of body weight per minute and this figure is referred to as VO2 Max. A world class rider would typically have a VO2 in the range of 75–90ml/kg/min compared to a typical Cat 3 rider who will be around 50ml/kg/min. Although VO2 Max is trainable to an extent and can also be improved by controlled weight loss, your upper limit is probably genetically predetermined.

What it feels like: Hard, really hard. You'll really be having to focus and both legs and lungs will be burning. No talking at this intensity, a grunt is probably all you'll be able to manage!

When you'd be in this zone: Hard efforts and intervals lasting between 3 and 8 minutes. During longer sessions, you could hit this zone attacking a short and steep climb but it'll take a lot out of you. When training for the Tour of Flanders sportive, with its steep cobbled climbs, I threw plenty of these efforts into my long rides.

ZONE 6: ANAEROBIC CAPACITY

Once you're pushing this hard, your body is having to produce energy without oxygen, or 'anaerobically'. Anaerobic capacity refers to the total amount of energy you're able to produce in this way.

What it feels like: A 100 per cent all-out sprint effort.

When you'd be in this zone: During sprints and high-intensity interval work. Efforts can be as short as 5 seconds but up to a minute. You wouldn't use heart rate for this intensity as it'll lag behind the effort too much. Just go for it full bore!

'SWEET SPOT'

There's an extra training zone, known as 'sweet spot', which I'll refer to in the ride and workout plans (see Chapter 4). Covering mid Zone 3 to mid Zone 4, it's a very beneficial zone for riders to train in. It's hard enough to elicit gains in FT but not as challenging and exhausting as full-on threshold work. This means you can train in your sweet spot and still recover to put in some decent efforts the following day or even later in the same ride. This makes it especially useful for commute training and for spicing up endurance rides. It can also be good for in-season maintenance training when you don't want to build excessive fatigue in your legs.

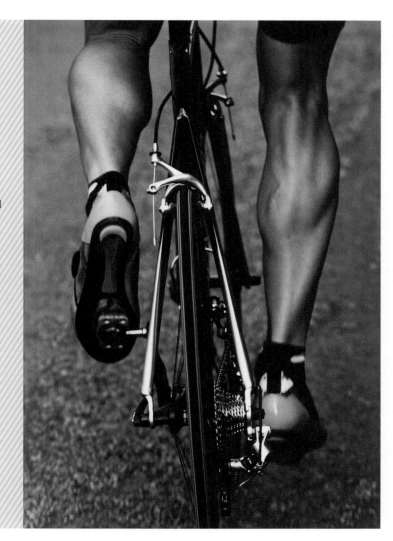

▶ For time pressed riders, the 'sweet spot' is an effective go-to training zone.

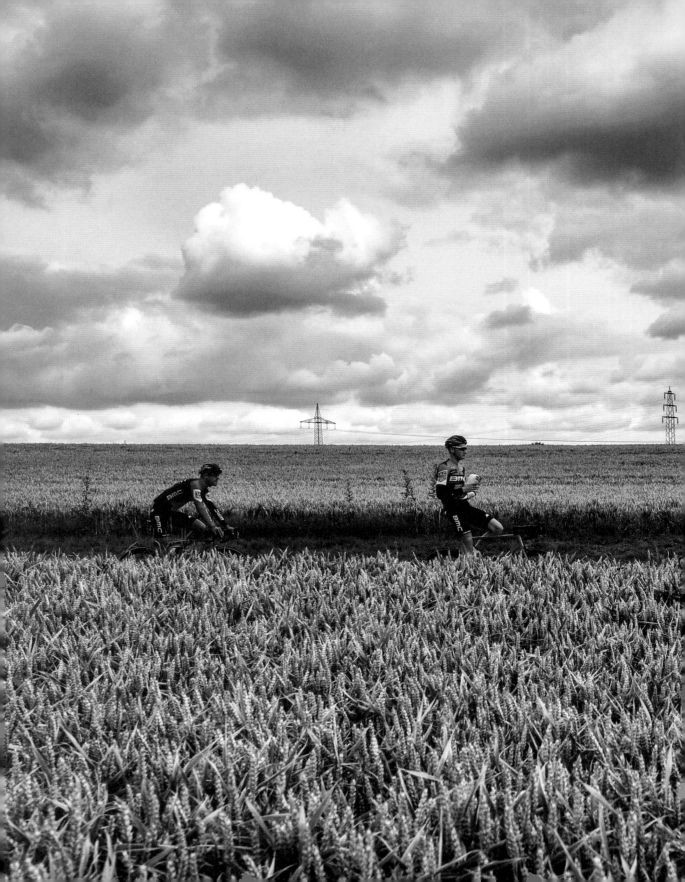

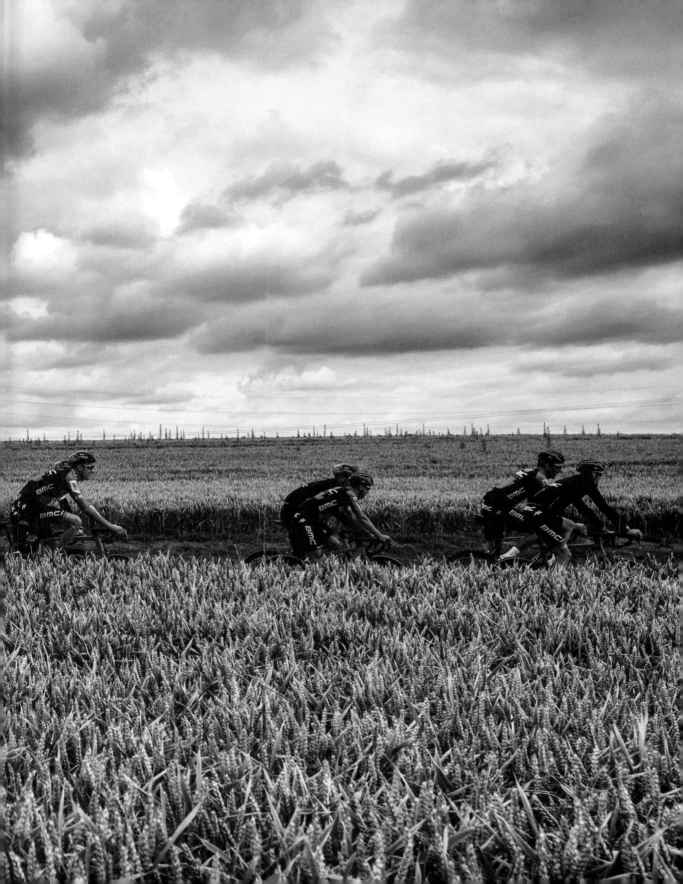

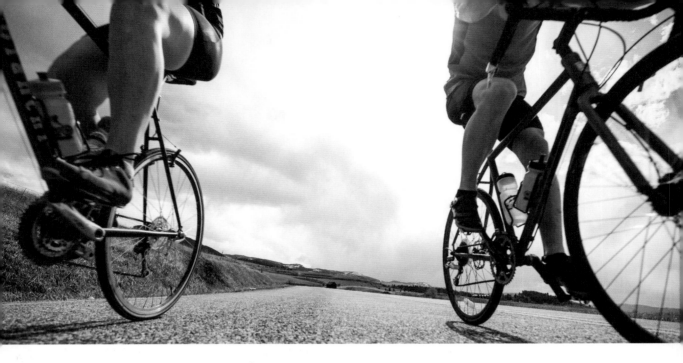

Testing indoors and outdoors

Now that you are aware of the importance of testing for FT, it is only fair to let you in on some bad news: you're probably going to have to do the test twice as there's typically a discrepancy between the values you'd observe out on the road and the values you'd achieve on an indoor trainer. In the last chapter, we talked about how useful and important an indoor trainer is for building cycling fitness. As using one will probably form a key component of your training, it's important that your training zones when using it are accurate.

It is important to be aware that, unfortunately, most riders find that their FT can differ considerably between outdoors and indoors. The difference tends to be more pronounced when training with heart rate. When riding indoors, riders' self-perception of the effort they're making will often be above what their heart rate is showing. There are a number of possible reasons for this, such as less use of the muscles in your upper body and trunk for balance lowering heart rate, overheating raising perception of effort, and just the boredom and lower motivation of training indoors. Riders will often see a downward shift in their zones by 10 beats per minute or more and attempting to train to your higher outdoors zones will result in incomplete sessions and frustration. Power users usually see less of a difference, especially if they have decent fans and are able to stay cool, but the sheer psychological challenge of pushing hard indoors can result in lower values.

In light of this, it is advised to test for FT and set zones for indoors and outdoors. You may find that the results are fairly close and, if within 5bpm or 10 watts, you can probably work with the same zones. Don't forget that you'll need to schedule in a rest day before both tests, but they're great stand-alone workouts anyway.

Retesting

Training zones are not static and should change as your fitness develops. If you're training with power and testing for FTP, you should see this value creeping up as you gain fitness.

For heart rate users, the gains aren't quite as tangible. With training, FTHR can go up, drop or even remain static. This can be confusing and even demotivating but it's important to remember that FTHR, unlike FTP, isn't a measure of 'fitness'. FTHR is just how hard your heart is beating when you're riding at your threshold, it's not a measure of the speed or power you're producing. It's still important to test regularly for it, as any changes can result in your training zones shifting significantly. If you can accurately replicate test conditions, only probably possible on an indoor trainer, you can also record average speed or distance covered and this could give a better indicator of changes in your fitness.

Whether training with heart rate or power, you should aim to retest for threshold every 8–12 weeks. It's important that you're well rested before testing so allow at least one recovery day before it and ideally schedule testing at the beginning of a week that follows a recovery week.

◀ It's not unusual to have to test for and set zones for both outdoor and indoor training.

Common problems with training to zones
Sticking to Zone 2

Many riders who are new to monitoring their intensity when riding and training to zones struggle to stay in the lower zones. This particularly applies to heart rate users and riding in Zones 1 and 2 during endurance sessions. They find they have to make a real effort to slow down in order to stop their heart rate creeping up into Zone 3 and even 4. Understandably they find this frustrating, especially when they see they're riding their regular routes slower or are being dropped by their ridemates. The problem stems from that 'physiological no-man's-land' that I mentioned at the start of the chapter. For many riders it can feel like a comfortable and sustainable pace, but the reality is that it's not. It can be okay for 1, 2 or even 3 hours, especially if there's a leisurely café stop at some point, but if you try to ride at that intensity for a long continuous sportive or training ride, you'll find yourself blowing up and significantly slowing down later in the ride.

For sportives, Zone 2 is your default riding intensity on the flat and you have to train your body to be able to function in it. Fail to do this and you'll never fulfil your cycling potential. In Zone 2 you're able to take on and process carbohydrates and, if you're well trained at riding at that intensity, also utilise your body's fat reserves. This means that you're able to maintain your body's carbohydrate supply and keep riding strongly. This especially applies when the road kicks up; you're forced to up your effort into Zones 3 and 4 for the climb and, at that intensity, you'll be almost totally reliant on carbohydrates. If you ride in Zones 3 and 4 predominately or haven't invested time in training your body to perform in Zone 2, you won't be tapping into your body's fat reserves and will be rapidly burning through your body's limited carbohydrate supplies. At that intensity, you won't be able to properly process the fuel you take on to replenish those supplies and, even if you could, the maximum you can use – about 90g (3oz) per hour – isn't enough to fuel your effort without the help of those fat reserves. Your carbohydrate supplies steadily dwindle as the ride goes on and, although you may feel fine, it's a ticking time bomb. Eventually, usually on a climb in the fourth or fifth hour, you come to a grinding halt.

Although it can be hard and frustrating at first, you have to be disciplined at sticking to those lower zones for the key endurance rides. Developing your fitness at this key Zone 2 intensity forms the foundations of being a successful endurance cyclist and can't be skipped. The good news is that after 8–12 weeks of structured training to zones, most riders find that their bodies adapt and their pace and ability to ride in Zone 2 significantly improves. During that adaptive phase, however, especially if you're a Zone 3 cruiser, there are a number of steps you can take to make the process a bit easier.

PICK YOUR ROUTES ACCORDINGLY It's much easier to control your heart rate or power if the route is flat. If a session calls for extended periods of riding in Zone 2, try to avoid the hills.

FIT LOWER GEARS If hills are unavoidable, fit some really low gears and don't feel embarrassed about spinning up even the gentlest incline.

RIDE IN A GROUP Riding in a group and following the wheel of another rider can reduce the effort by up to 30 per cent. Explain to the riders you're with what you're trying to achieve from the ride and that you're not just shirking your pull on the front.

RIDE SOLO Conversely, sometimes riding in a group can bring out that competitive spirit and you may find yourself goaded into riding harder than you want. If this is the case, or your ego just doesn't allow you to ease up and let the group go, a block of solo training might be a good idea.

CARBOHYDRATE-FASTED TRAINING Carbohydrate-fasted training can help to develop your body's ability to burn fat as a fuel and so improve your efficiency and ability to stay in lower zones. We'll talk more about carbohydrate-fasted training, and how and when to do it, in Chapter 4.

CHECK YOUR ZONES Double-check that you've calculated your zones correctly – you wouldn't be the first cyclist to struggle with maths! There's also the possibility that your FTP/FTHR result was inaccurate, although it's a fairly robust test and protocol. If you were tired or had an underlying illness, it's possible that you may not

▶ If you're struggling sticking to the lower training zones, riding in a group can definitely help.

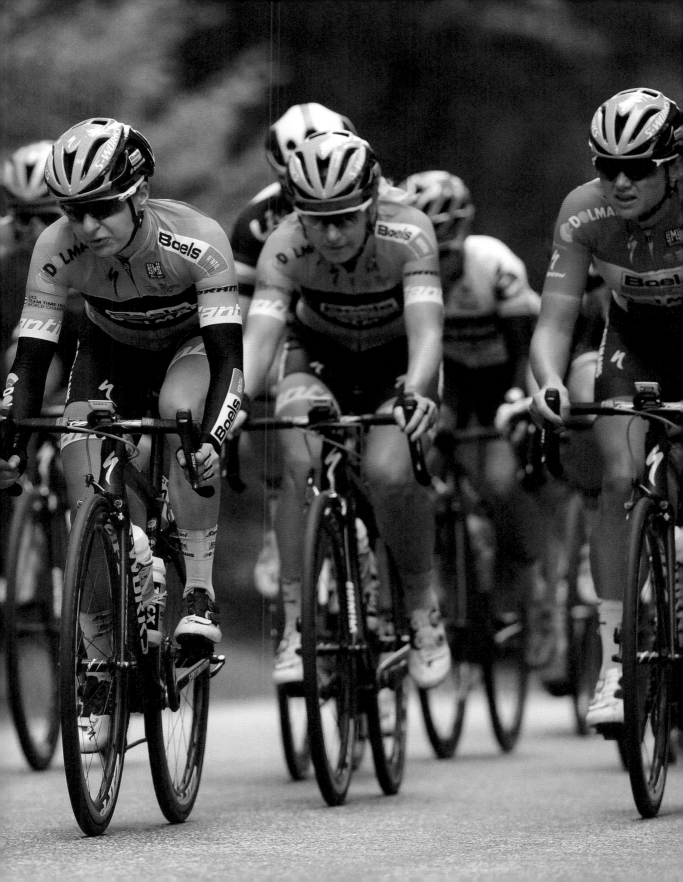

have been able to give it your all or that your heart rate was suppressed. This could produce a low result and correspondingly low-skewed training zones. Also, if it's your first time performing such a test, you might not have got the pacing right and not quite emptied the tank. If you suspect this might be the case, you can repeat the test. The more familiar you become with the test, the more accurate it becomes.

Relying on averages

One big mistake that riders new to training to zones often make is to rely on average heart rate or power. They'll see that a session requires 2 hours in Zone 2 but will go out and ride with barely a glance at their computer. They get home, download their ride data and see their average heart rate or power bang in the middle of Zone 2, job done. The problem is, it's possible to achieve such an average, especially if a route is hilly, having spent hardly any time in the target zone. On the climbs, they may have been battering themselves in Zones 4 or 5 but then, on the descents, freewheeling in Zone 1. So despite what the average showed, there was no riding in the target zone and none of the training and physiological objectives of the session have been achieved. A good analogy is a man standing with one foot in a bucket of ice and the other in a bucket of boiling water. Is he averagely comfortable?

You have to be constantly aware of and monitoring your intensity throughout the ride or effort. Set your computer to show zones, current wattage or heart rate and make sure you look at it and adjust your intensity to what it's showing. Power meter users will probably find it easier to display 3-second average power as this tends to fluctuate far less and is easier to ride to than current power. With experience, you'll soon develop a feel for your zones and an occasional glance will suffice.

Paralysis by analysis

A big problem, especially for power meter users, is that you can find yourself faced with a huge and bewildering amount of ride data. There's no doubting that power meters are incredibly powerful training tools and that we're only just scratching the surface of the power and pedalling analysis that they allow. However, although I strongly advise all riders to consider buying one, you don't need to spend hours looking at power data files to gain a lot of benefit from using one. Simply testing for FTP regularly, using it to set accurate training zones and then learning how to use them to accurately pace your riding will massively improve the performance of most riders. With time, you'll want to take advantage of additional metrics, such as Training Stress Score (TSS), which gives an objective rating of how hard a session was, and use more sophisticated session analysis and planning tools such as TrainingPeaks and GoldenCheetah. However, don't think you have to spend hours learning how to use a power meter and understand all of the metrics and data before you can start using one. If you're spending more time planning or analysing workouts than actually riding, you're getting it badly wrong.

Being a slave to the numbers

Training and riding to zones is essential if you want to get the most out of your cycling and, for the majority of your rides, you should know what you want to achieve and the zones you should be focusing on to achieve it. However, it's also important to remember why you started cycling, to occasionally leave the heart rate monitor or power meter at home and just to ride for pleasure. Whether it's in the off season or during a break from structured training, not all rides have to be training. The Sunday club run probably isn't the place for you to be riding to your numbers either. You'll either end up driving up the pace of the group or constantly slowing it down as you try to stick to your zones, neither of which is going to make you very popular. Also, if you're in a race situation, sometimes riding to your numbers can limit both your performance and your ability to react to the race. In a circuit race, you're not going to bail out of a break just because your power meter is telling you you've exceeded the amount of time you can hold Zone 5 for! Although invaluable for pacing time trials, I'll sometimes tape over my power meter and ride to feel instead. I've set PBs doing this and, when I've checked my data after the event, found out that I needed to bump up my FTP and zones.

How to improve your cycling performance

Monitor intensity

If you don't already use a heart rate monitor or power meter, you're severely limiting your likelihood of progressing as a cyclist. Without them you're effectively riding blind and wasting valuable time in the saddle.

Test for FTP/FTHR

Testing for your FTP/FTHR is the essential and unavoidable first step to effective training and reaching your cycling potential. Relying on inaccurate generic formulae or zone auto calculate functions is a shortcut that will mean all subsequent training is fundamentally flawed.

Test indoors and outdoors

Some riders find that their FTHR and even FTP can vary depending on whether it's tested on an indoor trainer or out on the road. Test for both and set two sets of training zones.

Retest regularly

Ensure you retest FTP/FTHR every 8–12 weeks. Don't worry too much what your FTHR does, it's not an indicator of fitness. Although it's a test, it's still a great workout and shouldn't be thought of as a missed session.

Be disciplined

Once you know your zones, stick to them. This applies to hitting high zones in hard sessions and riding in lower zones during steadier, endurance-focused workouts.

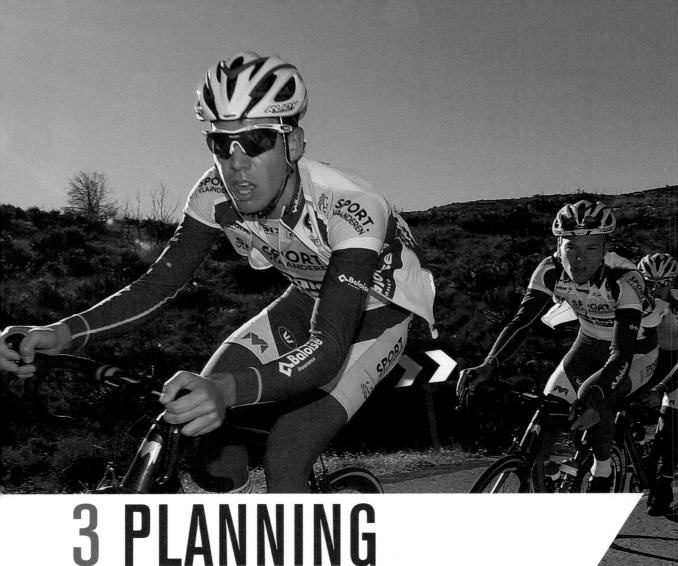

3 PLANNING YOUR TRAINING

WITHOUT STRUCTURE AND PLANNING YOU'LL NEVER PERFORM TO YOUR BEST. IN THIS CHAPTER LEARN HOW TO PLAN YOUR YEAR AROUND KEY EVENTS, INCLUDING SPECIFIC TRAINING BLOCKS AND STRUCTURING YOUR TRAINING WEEKS.

'I inherited that calm from my father, who was a farmer. You sow, you wait for good or bad weather, you harvest, but working is something you always need to do.'

MIGUEL INDURAIN, FIVE-TIME TOUR DE FRANCE WINNER

FOR ALL PROFESSIONAL RIDERS, one of the key moments of their year is when they sit down with their directeur sportif and are handed their race schedule for the year. This will dictate their existence for the next 12 months and determine their training structure and priorities. A Classics specialist, such as Greg van Avermaet, will be looking for early season form for gruelling spring races such as the Paris–Roubaix and the Tour of Flanders. As the focus changes to the hillier Ardennes Classics (Amstel Gold, La Flèche Wallonne and Liège–Bastogne–Liège), punchier climbers, like Philippe Gilbert, start to appear, and the odd Grand Tour contender – especially if they have the Giro d'Italia in mind – may even make a cameo appearance, but will rarely trouble the podium.

In the modern era, genuine Tour de France contenders have focused solely on those three weeks in July. They'll loiter at the back of the field, building up racing mileage during a few early season events, such as the Tour Down Under. They'll then usually disappear off the racing scene and dedicate themselves to a monk-like training existence – at the top of Mount Teide on Tenerife if you're Chris Froome –

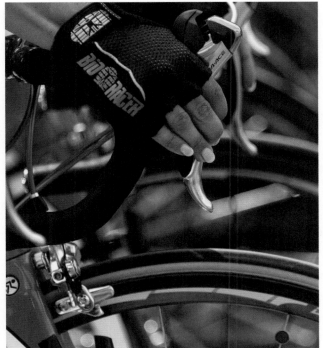

▼ No matter what your level, planning your riding year is an essential part of improving your cycling performance.

before emerging for pre-Tour final tune-up events, such as the Dauphiné Libéré, in full Tour-winning form. This approach relies on structured and methodical training, rather than chaotic and often unpredictable racing, to deliver Tour contenders to the Grand Départ in the best form possible. From the moment after crossing the finish line on the Champs Élysées at the previous year's race, the next 11 months are meticulously planned into dedicated training blocks.

Similarly, goal focused training and planning back from key events has been one of the pillars of success of the Great Britain Cycling Team. This approach began with timed events, such as the team pursuit, kilo and team sprint, on the track. With such controlled events and environment, it was a relatively simple calculation to determine the power output needed by each rider to set a world-beating time and how long they had to get the riders there.

'For the Rio 2016 Olympics things focused down from two years out when we sat down with our team coach, physiologist and strength/conditioning coach and they presented a plan to us called What it Takes to Win. This was the time that they thought we'd have to ride to win gold in the team pursuit at the Olympics and the power we'd have to achieve to do that. This was then broken down into smaller performance goals. These markers would be used to track improvement along the way. We'd then use a phase planner with all the competitions in the lead up to the Olympics.' **KATIE ARCHIBALD**, GREAT BRITAIN CYCLING TEAM

This 'What it Takes to Win?' philosophy was famously applied to the far less controllable environment of road racing for Mark Cavendish's win at the 2011 World Championships in Copenhagen. It doesn't always go 100 per cent to plan, though. For the 2012 Olympic road race, detailed calculations were made regarding Cavendish's required power-to-weight ratio to keep him in touch during the multiple ascents of Box Hill.

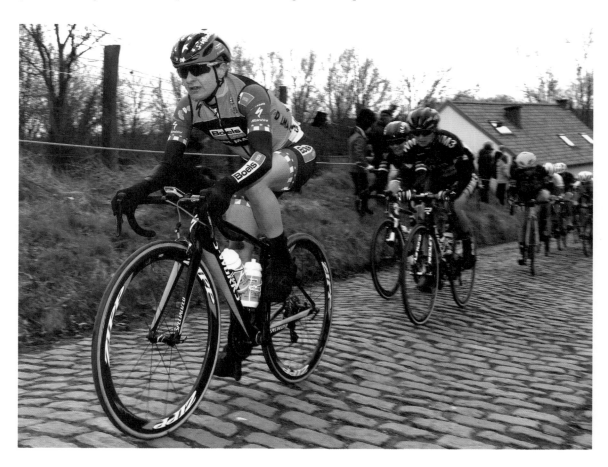

'Planning a season is a joint effort between the directeur sportif, coaches and the rider. It's then a case of seeing how that fits in with the other riders and working out a plan. Once the plan is in place and we've decided which races I'm targeting we can plan the racing blocks and when I need to peak. However, things rarely go to plan. For the last two seasons we've had injuries and illnesses within the team, so we've had to be flexible and adapt. It's all about communication and being adaptable.'

TIFFANY CROMWELL, CANYON/SRAM

However, despite being in the form of his life, race tactics conspired to find him not part of the medal-deciding finale on the Mall. The controllables had been controlled but sometimes the vagaries and unpredictable nature of bike racing confound even the most rigorous planning, preparation and sports science. However, it's undeniable that everything that could have been done had been done to put Mark Cavendish in with the best possible chance of winning that Olympic gold medal.

◄ Identify the specific demands of your target event and tailor your training towards them.

For the ultimate example of targeting and working back from a key event, you have to return to the Great British Cycling Team track riders and their four-yearly appointment with the Olympic Games. After the success of London 2012, many of the riders appeared to go into a competitive hibernation, and although there was the odd rainbow jersey or World Cup win, the dominance that had been seen at the London 2012 velodrome seemed to have vanished. Yes, notable riders such as Sir Chris Hoy and Victoria Pendleton had retired but younger riders, such as double gold medallist Jason Kenny, seemed to be dwelling in the doldrums of competitive mediocrity. Even in the final World Championships, six months before the 2016 Rio Games, the Great Britain squad looked distinctly below par. To the outside observer, coming anywhere near the 2012 medal haul looked extremely unlikely. However, once the racing started in Rio, with a dominating performance in the team sprint, it was obvious that the Great Britain Cycling Team were back to their world-beating best. Much was made about new tech, equipment and marginal gains, but the main factor behind the success was single-minded focus, planning and a four-year cycle with the Olympic Games as the clear and only goal. Many other nations had chosen to try to 'double peak' their riders, hitting top form for both the World Championships and the Olympics. However, to achieve this would have involved a taper, a planned easing back of training before an event, which, despite meaning victories at the World Championships, also meant lost training time in that crucial final build-up to Rio. The British team trained right through the World Championships, accepting that they wouldn't be at their peak but knowing they were banking valuable weeks of hard training that their rivals were missing out on. They'd been applying this approach, not just during the Olympic year, but throughout the preceding three years. Those weeks of not fully tapering for every World Championships or World Cup added up to maybe months of extra training. When they did finally fully taper into the Olympics, they reaped the rewards of that patience and planning.

Whether you're targeting a big sportive, a particular time trial or the start of the race season, assessing the demands of your event, working out what it will take for you to succeed and then constructing a realistic and effective training plan is essential. Only by applying structure to your training can you ensure that your fitness is progressing, that you're maximising your gains from the time you have and that you'll be in peak condition for your target event.

The fundamentals of training

There are three basic interrelated requirements of any structured training plan. The first is that it has to provide the body with overload to stimulate adaptation. Our bodies are hardwired by millions of years of evolution to preserve energy and not to invest our valuable reserves into costly endeavours, such as building muscle, unless we give

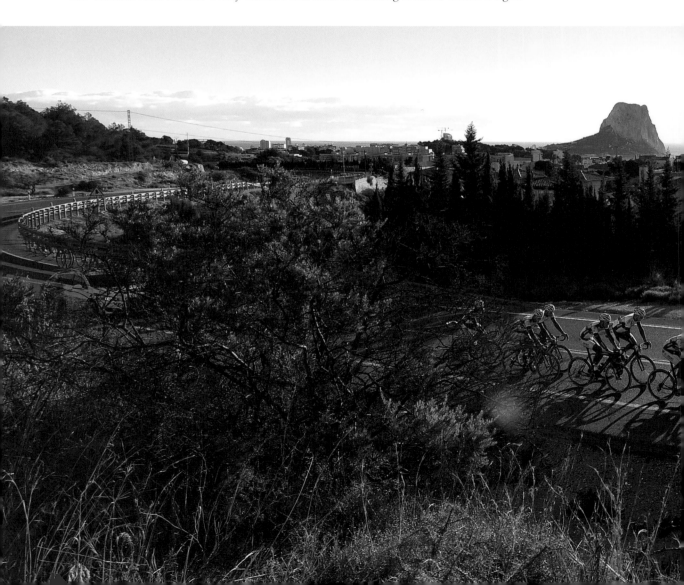

them a good reason to. You have to keep raising the bar and that's why, if you keep doing the same training week in and week out, you'll eventually hit a plateau and stop improving.

The next requirement is that the overload has to be progressive. That bar has to be incrementally raised over time, not suddenly and dramatically elevated by 'get fit quick' or panicked crash training.

The final classic requirement of a training plan is specificity. Simply put, the best training for any activity is doing that activity. To get better at cycling, you have to cycle. It sounds obvious, but often gets ignored. This fundamental of training does come with a major caveat, though, which will be covered further in Chapter 5 when we discuss 'off the bike' training. There's an increasing body of evidence that off the bike conditioning, such as strength and mobility work, can benefit cycling performance. More importantly, it challenges the body outside of the very limited and fixed movement patterns of cycling. This makes you more robust and resilient,

▼ Make sure you always consider the fundamentals of training when devising your plan.

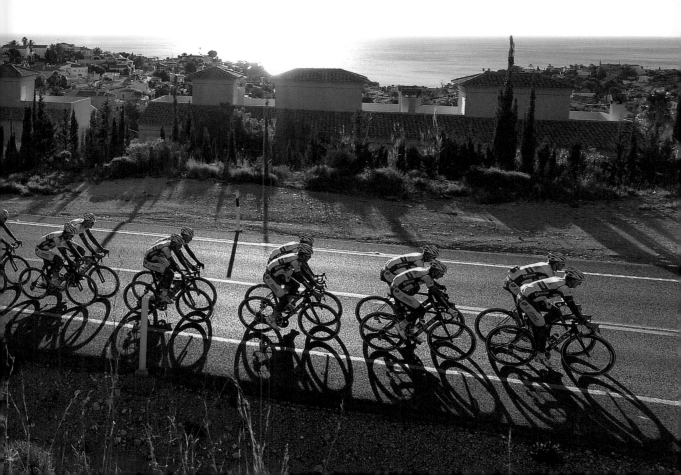

and less likely to pick up injuries in day-to-day life. Professional cycling teams have really embraced off the bike conditioning in recent years, realising the benefits to rider health, career longevity and on the bike performance.

'I think it's really important to do some off the bike training, such as weights, but more for health than performance. Through October to November I'd always do a lot of work in the gym and, despite sticking at 4–5 per cent body fat, would put on 5lb of muscle. I'd worry about the extra weight but it always fell off and I'd always still manage to peak too early in the spring! However, despite numerous crashes, I never really got injured and my bone density and blood values were always good. I credit that partly to luck and genetics, and partly to the gym work every off-season.'

PHIL GAIMON, EX-PRO WITH GARMIN-SHARP AND CANNONDALE-DRAPAC

For riders whose job isn't riding their bike, it's probably even more important as you'll have more non-riding demands placed on your body. If you hurt yourself gardening, carrying shopping or lifting your children out of the car, that's time off the bike. You have to ensure that you schedule in enough cycling but also make sure you don't neglect off the bike training.

In addition to these three fundamentals, there are three more areas that have to be considered and factored into any training plan. The first is that both the end goal and the training plan have to be realistic. A goal should challenge you but it has to be attainable within the confines of your ability and the amount of time you can dedicate to training. The same applies to your training plan. Avoid scheduling an amount of training that's right on the upper limit of what your life allows. It's inevitable that you'll end up missing sessions, which can often lead to becoming demotivated and falling completely off the training wagon.

Next is that your training has to be consistent. This is related to both progression and overload and means that you can't be a binge or sporadic trainer. The physiological adaptations that result in improved endurance fitness take time and a consistency of training to occur. One week, one month or arguably even one year of consistent training doesn't make a great cyclist. A study on professional cyclists found that their efficiency of pedal stroke boiled down to one simple variable: the number of pedal strokes and miles they'd performed to that point.

Finally, but arguably most importantly, is the key aspect of recovery. I'll talk more about the importance of recovery, how to optimise it and the ramifications of neglecting it in Chapter 7 but, without adequate recovery, you'll never progress as a cyclist. After providing a training stimulus, it's as the body recovers that it adapts and becomes stronger. Being able to complete all of the workouts you have scheduled is only part of the training plan equation. If you're unable to also schedule in adequate recovery time, the training plan is severely flawed. Top-level full-time cyclists are brilliant at recovery. Being able to dedicate the time they're not riding to recovery is the factor — probably more so than the training they do — that elevates them above riders who are having to balance training with another full-time occupation. Getting

▶ Hard work on the bike is important but it has to be balanced by recovery off it.

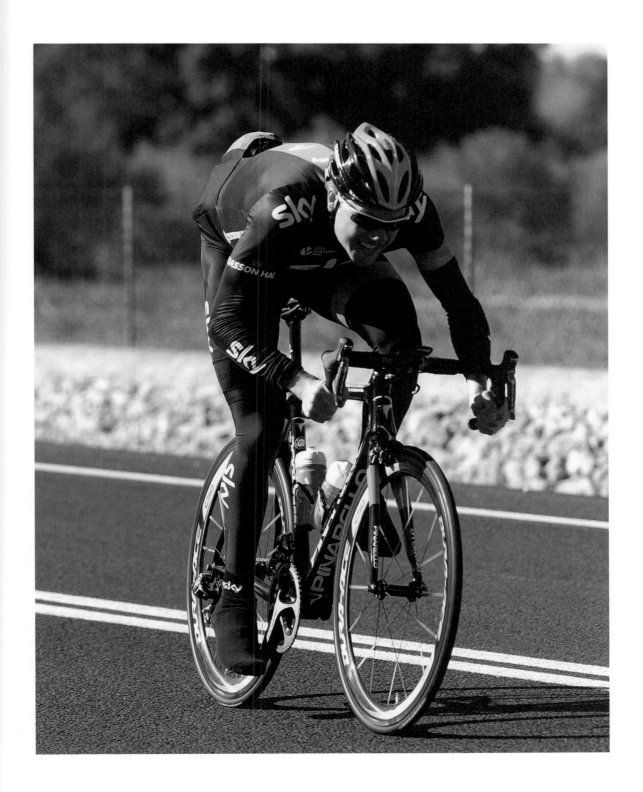

WE'RE ALL INDIVIDUALS

One area of sports science that's receiving a lot of attention is the needs, requirements and characteristics of the individual athlete. What's becoming realised and accepted is that we all react and respond differently to training stimuli and that a 'one size fits all' approach to training is far from optimal. Some athletes are able to tolerate huge training loads, gain fitness fast and maintain peaks of form for extended periods. These so-called 'responders' are undoubtedly genetically blessed but the exact mechanisms that confer these abilities on them are only just starting to be revealed. When you were at school, there was probably a child in your class (you might have been lucky and it was you) who was just brilliant at everything. Such a child would probably be a responder. Being able to recognise such responders will be the future of talent identification programmes. They won't be looking for the young athletes currently producing the best numbers on a testing rig, as they might already have peaked. They'll be searching for those who have the greatest potential to develop and handle training load.

Former Great Britain Cycling Team lead physiotherapist Phil Burt talks in terms of macro-absorbers and micro-adjusters. Macro-absorbers are the riders who are able to cope with huge training and racing loads and, in the event of having to swap onto a spare bike, not be fazed by a less than optimal set-up. He cites Geraint Thomas as a prime example of a macro-adjuster. He soaks up training, rarely gets injured and has ridden half a stage of the Tour de France on a teammate's spare bike. It's more than likely that Geraint Thomas is a classic responder. On the flip side, Phil uses Ben Swift as an example of a micro-adjuster. He'll notice the smallest change to his bike set-up, is more prone to niggles and has to be far more aware of how he schedules his training and racing. Both have become incredibly successful riders but have to approach their cycling very differently.

The gains that two athletes can expect from following an identical training plan can be very different and just because a particular training plan has worked for a friend or clubmate, it doesn't mean that it will work or is optimal for you. The guidelines in this book provide a solid grounding for constructing your own structured training plan, but it's important to realise that they'll have to be tailored to your own specific needs and physiology. Don't be afraid to experiment on yourself and try to develop a strong sense of body awareness. If you're feeling tired, struggling for motivation or not making the progress you expected, don't just keep ploughing on regardless. Stop, re-evaluate objectively and adjust your training accordingly.

◄ Just like your bike set-up, your training has to be specific to your individual needs.

out of the 'more is more' mindset and shifting the emphasis from quantity of training to the quality of training and recovery is probably one of the most significant positive steps you can take. If you don't recover from a workout, you won't reap the rewards from it and it'll impact on the quality of the next and subsequent sessions. Neglect it in the long term and you risk not only diminishing performance but the demotivation, illness and injury risks that are associated with overtraining syndrome. Don't forget, along with the training sessions you do, work, family life and other activities all contribute to your total 'training load' and have to be accounted for.

> 'I was very good at resting and recovery when I was a full-time rider. If I felt as though I needed a day off, it would literally be the whole day horizontal on the sofa watching TV. It was absolute 100 per cent rest. As my career progressed, more things came into my life, house, marriage, children, and it was the recovery side of my training that suffered.'
>
> **DEAN DOWNING**, EX-PRO, FORMER BRITISH CIRCUIT RACE CHAMPION AND NOW COACH

Demands of your event

If you're targeting a particular event, what does it involve and do you have any specific goals or expectations? If you're targeting a mountainous Alpine sportive such as L'Étape, your training needs will differ significantly from those of a rider who's aiming to tackle the cobbled climbs of the Tour of Flanders. Both riders will require a solid endurance base to be able to ride for 6 hours or more but you will want to focus on longer efforts and intervals around your FTP/FTHR to prepare for the 20km-plus (12 mile) climbs you'll face in the Alps. For the relatively short but brutally steep cobbled climbs of Flanders, the emphasis will be more on shorter but higher intensity Zone 5 efforts and the ability to recover from them. Doing some research into the demands of your chosen event and replicating those demands in training is essential if you want to meet your goals.

A great example of tailoring yourself and your training to the demands of your event can be seen if you look at the career of Sir Bradley Wiggins. When he made the transition for Olympic track rider to Tour de France winner, he dropped in the region of 10kg and focused on developing his ability on long climbs as opposed to higher octane track efforts. Then, when he targeted the 2014 time trial World Championships, he and his team realised that he needed to change his morphology and physiology significantly from the stripped-down and lightweight Tour de France winning rider of 2012. The 47km Ponferrada course required more raw power and so a block of strength work, muscle gain and higher intensity efforts followed. With a return to the track for his hour record and Rio, those new goals required even more strength and power. Throughout his career it's been a case of identifying what it would take to win, and adapting both himself and his training to work towards that specific goal.

'The directeur sportif decides which races the team will be doing and which riders he ideally wants at them. He'll then come to me and check that the riders he's selected for the races are best suited to it physiologically and will be ready for it. If there's a key race, say the Tour of Flanders, for the riders who we want contesting that race, we'll schedule their training and other races to ensure that they peak for that event. It's always a three-way collaboration between the directeur sportif, the coach/physiologist and, of course, the rider.

Once the races are in place, we'll then tend to plan training in 4-week blocks. You have to listen to your body and adapt your training accordingly. It's a constant cycle of communication and feedback from the rider about how they're feeling, we adjust their training based on that and then plan the next five or six days.'

ANDREAS LANG, TEAM PHYSIOLOGIST, CANYON/SRAM

Planning your year

Once you have identified your target events, you can start planning your year. This doesn't mean spending hours creating a highly detailed spreadsheet with every session set in stone but rather deciding what your priorities are throughout the year.

Work back from those key events. Allow 1 or 2 weeks immediately before them as a taper and then 8–10-week focused blocks leading into them. Depending on the event, you may also want to plan some downtime afterwards where you take some time out from structured training. Avoid the temptation to pack in too many target events. You can back a couple of them up and, for shorter league-style racing such as time trials, crits, track league and cyclo-cross, compete on a weekly basis; but if you're tackling 'A' category events – big sportives or multi-day rides – and want to give them your best, you'll only be able to schedule in a few each year. If you find there are too many events that you want to do, assign 'B' or 'C' status to some of them. You'll view these more as training events and, without tapering down fully for them, not expect to perform to your best but still get valuable miles in your legs and event day experience.

Depending on the sort of events you prefer, you'll probably find that you have an 'off season' where you have no events scheduled. For many riders this occurs during the winter but if, for example, you race cyclo-cross or indoor track, this might not be the case. I'd always recommend having 2–4 weeks off the bike, or at least off from structured training, at the start of your off season, probably following your final 'A' event of the season. You probably won't feel like it as you're likely to be on top form but, for longevity in the sport, avoiding boredom or burnout, firing up your energy

▶ You can't perform at your best 52 weeks a year. Identify and plan your training around certain key events.

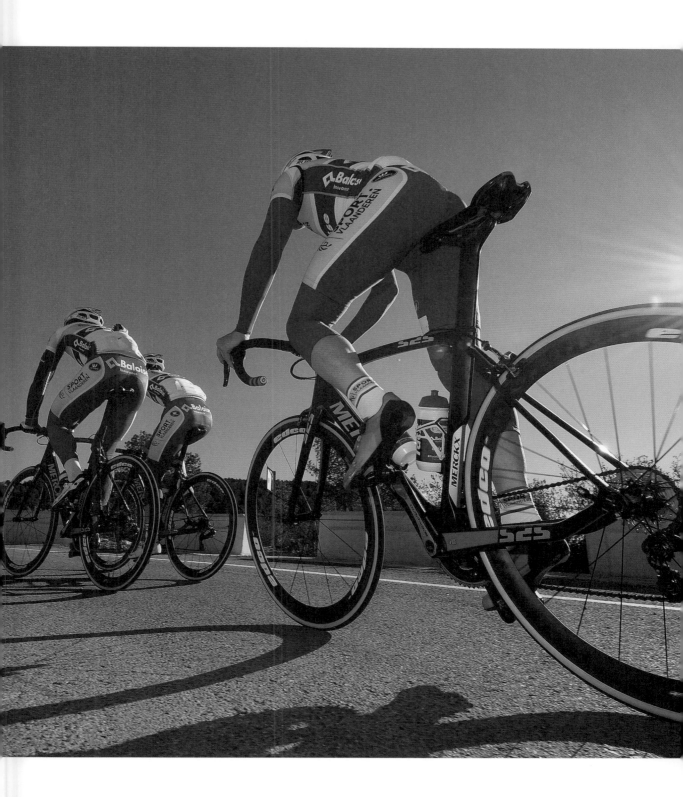

and enthusiasm before the grind of off-season training and for family harmony, try to schedule in it. Use some of this time to look back on the season just gone and to assess what went well, what could be improved upon, your strengths and your weaknesses. How did you train during the previous off season and what could be improved on?

The off season is where you'll be looking to focus primarily on building your endurance base. This doesn't mean just grinding out slow miles as, especially for non-professional riders, keeping some intensity in your riding is the best way to maximise training gains from your relatively limited time on the bike. You will, however, be aiming to get some long rides in, work on longer intervals on the turbo to raise FTP and probably also including some focused off the bike work to develop mobility and strength. Your top end fitness may drop off a bit and, especially if it's the winter, you may gain a bit of insulation. Gaining a few pounds over the winter is no bad thing as it'll help you feel the cold less on long rides and can give your immune system a bit of a helping hand. Avoid gaining too much, though, or you'll be forced to try and crash it off in the spring. This can be difficult and combining calorie restriction with higher intensity training can compromise your training gains. If your fitness is analogous to building a house, you're laying the foundations for the subsequent floors of the pre-season and season to come. It's a commonly used cliché but, in all endurance sports, winter miles mean summer smiles. Neglect your off-season foundation building and every subsequent layer of fitness is compromised. Be disciplined about your off-season training and be clear what you want to achieve. As much as getting out and riding in the cold, wet and dark, this discipline also applies to sticking to the training zones and goals of the sessions that'll lay down solid foundations. Every club has a rider who rips up the club runs through the off season but never features when the real racing starts. Don't be that rider. You can't hold peak form through the entire year and, if you squander it during the off season, you'll never perform when it really matters.

The pre-season, usually late winter and early spring, is when you start to up the intensity as you transition from training to racing and target events. Volume will generally start to come down, but not necessarily if it's a long event you're aiming for, and more intensity and higher-level efforts will be introduced. If you've been lifting weights for off the bike conditioning during the off season, you'll probably reduce the number of sessions from two or three down to two or even one. The goal will be to maintain the strength you've gained rather than build more and, by removing some of the resistance training load on your legs, they should feel sharper and more capable of higher intensity efforts. You might also decide to enter some early season events to test your legs and see where you are. In the UK, 'Hardrider' time trials take place on hilly and technical courses through February and March and are great for seeing how your off season has gone. You'll find similar early-season events in most other countries and, although you may not be in peak form, they're definitely worth seeking out.

Into the season you're really putting the roof on your house of fitness and doing general maintenance work. You should be focusing on minimising fatigue to maximise form in your build-up to target events and, if you have a significant gap between events, working on your perceived weaknesses where possible.

▶ Your training structure should continually change throughout the year, don't just do the same sessions week in week out.

SQUEEZING IN
ONE MORE EVENT

Sitting down and planning out your year and the events you want to target is exciting. It's probably the winter, you're feeling sluggish and slow, thinking ahead to having the sun on your back and being in racing shape, it's easy to get carried away. You'll identify your main target event for the year but, seeing that there's another brilliant one a few weeks later, figure you'll be able to carry your great form through and nail that one too. Unfortunately, and we all suffer from this blindness, you forget how hard you push yourself training for a big event, how much the day itself takes out of you and that, almost every time, you're ill or exhausted afterwards. I've lost count of the number of times I've done this, and every time I make the same mistake and waste another entry fee, I vow not to do it again. In 2016, my big target was the Track World Masters in October. Planning my year, I noticed that the League of Veteran Racers Track Championships was in late October and figured I'd be in amazing form from the Worlds. Well, the Worlds went brilliantly, winning a rainbow jersey in the Team Pursuit, but, painfully predictably, immediately afterwards I went down with a chest infection and had to pull out of the second event.

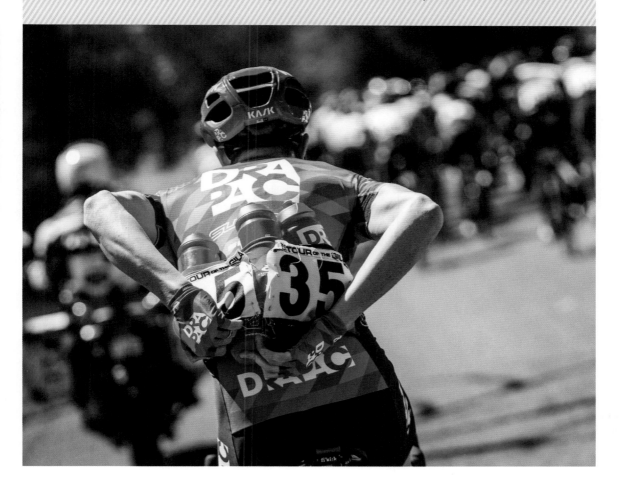

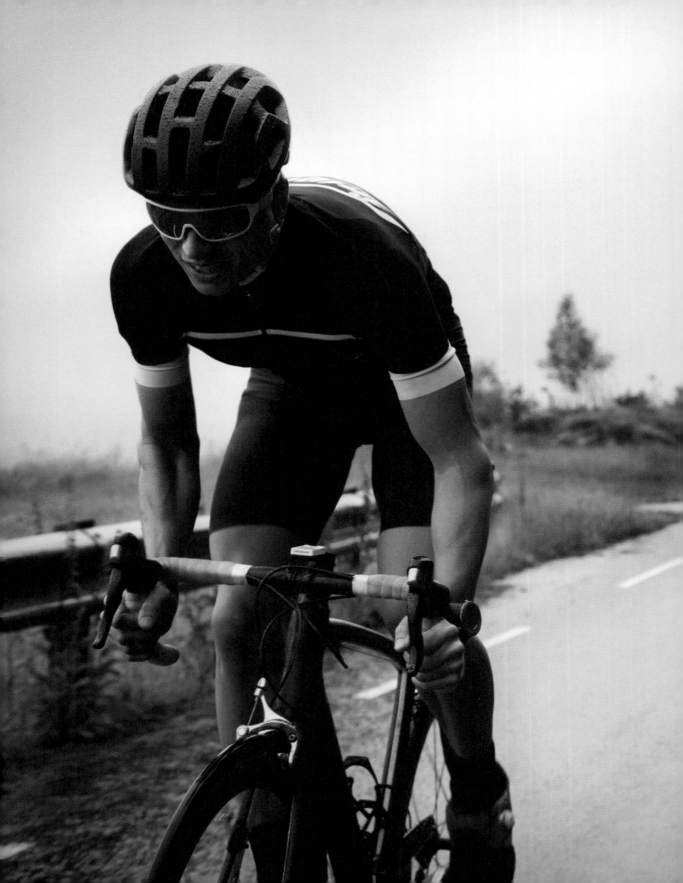

Planning a training block

Deciding on the length of your training blocks comes down to a number of factors. The first is that you have to give your body enough time and consistent training for physiological changes to occur. The exact length of time will depend on your individual physiology, psychology, your resilience to training load and the goal of the training block. You'll have to experiment with what works best for you but an average training block will generally be 8–12 weeks. I personally err towards 8 weeks. I'm a fairly fast responder and have a solid base of endurance fitness built over 16 years. I find, if I try to push on to 12 weeks, that progress will stall, I'll lose motivation and often get ill. When it comes to the target event, I'll be stale and will have given my best 4 or 5 weeks ago.

Once you've identified your block, you should then break it up into two or three smaller 4-week chunks. During each of these 4-week periods, you'll spend 3 weeks building training load by increasing volume, intensity or both. You'll then have a recovery week, when you'll drop training load. These recovery weeks are vital as it's during this time that your body adapts and you become fitter. Too many riders make the mistake of just exponentially ramping their training up week after week and not scheduling in regular recovery weeks. Although they'll initially make good progress, especially if starting from a relatively low fitness level, they will inevitably hit a plateau and even start to regress. They certainly won't be optimising their potential and, by driving their bodies into a state of non-functional overreaching or overtraining (concepts we'll discuss in Chapter 7), risk illness and injury.

For planning and recording training and seeing its impact, a huge advantage of using a power meter is that, for every ride, you can get an objective number for how stressful any ride was on your body. TrainingPeak is used by the Great Britain Cycling Team to plan and track the training of its riders and, if you're using a power meter, you should definitely consider signing up for an account. Known as Training Stress Score (TSS), your FTP is used to calculate the load of a session on your body. Duration, intensity and variability, such as during an interval session, all increase the TSS. As a reference point, an hour ridden evenly at FTP, theoretically the longest you could sustain that intensity, would score 100. By keeping a tally of your TSS, you can see exactly the training load you've accumulated. TrainingPeaks has a brilliant feature, its Performance Management Chart (PMC), which allows you to track and log TSS. Your TSS contributes to three lines on the chart. Acute Training Load (ATL) is the short-term effects of your workouts done in the last 7 days and is a reflection of your fatigue. Chronic Training Load (CTL) is the cumulative effect of training done in the last 42 days; this is your fitness. Training Stress Balance (TSB) is the difference between CTL and ATL from the previous day. This calculation of fitness minus fatigue is an indicator of your form. This shows why recovery weeks and tapers – easing back on training in the lead-up to a target event – are so important. Crucially, the PMC allows you to plot the TSS of future workouts, which is brilliant for optimising form for key events. Form and tapering used to be great mysteries but, with power meters and this type of analysis software, much of the guesswork is removed. Don't forget,

◄ Try to divide your year up into focused 8-12 week training blocks.

though, that no matter how good the data or analysis tools, we're not machines and we all respond differently to training. Use TSS and the PMC as a guide but don't be a slave to it or your power meter. Listen to your body and learn to use intuition as well as hard data to govern your training.

Even if you don't use a power meter, the components of TSS are very helpful to understand training load and how your body will respond to it. The load on your body of any session, and also accumulated load, is determined by duration, intensity and variability. This allows us to see why the traditional pro approach of massive volume low intensity training did, to a certain extent, work. Their training load was supplied purely by volume. Even with the time available to put in huge volumes of training, full-time riders now realise that by also factoring in more intensity and variability, by including high end efforts and intervals throughout the off-season, they can train in a far more effective way. For riders with limited time to train, this is even more relevant.

Whether you're training with power or heart rate, having accurate training zones is essential to the success of any training block. You should always schedule in an FT test at the beginning of any training block, remembering that you should have at least 24 hours of rest beforehand. I'd then recommend retesting at the beginning of Week 9 of any block, or the first week of your next block if it's an 8-week block, having had a recovery week beforehand. You should also retest FT if you've had any significant time off the bike or haven't managed to train consistently.

An example of a simple 12-week off-season training block, with an emphasis on endurance and strength, is given below (full session descriptions of the named workouts are given in Chapter 4).

12-WEEK OFF-SEASON TRAINING BLOCK

Week	Focus	Notes/Key sessions
1	Build 1	**FT test at start of week**, strength intervals and 3-hour endurance ride
2	Build 2	Strength intervals x2 and 3:30 endurance ride
3	Build 3	Strength intervals x2 and 4:00 endurance ride
4	Recovery	High cadence on rollers x2 and fun 2-hour MTB ride
5	Build 1	Strength intervals x2 and 4:00 endurance ride
6	Build 2	Strength intervals x2 and 4:30 endurance ride
7	Build 3	Strength intervals x2 and 5:00 endurance ride
8	Recovery	Strength intervals x2 and fun 2-hour MTB ride
9	Build 1	**FT test at start of week**, strength intervals and 4-hour endurance ride with tempo efforts
10	Build 2	Strength intervals x1, 2 x 20 mins sweet spot x1 and 4:30 endurance ride with tempo efforts
11	Build 3	Strength intervals x1, 2 x 20 mins sweet spot x1 and 5:00 endurance ride with tempo efforts
12	Recovery	High cadence on rollers x2 and fun MTB ride

Following the FT test at the start of Week 1, you can see how the endurance ride is increased over the following two weeks to add volume. The strength intervals session is a staple throughout this block, delivering on the bike strength training. One thing that you'll probably notice is that the sessions don't change much throughout the 12 weeks. Many riders, training plans and coaches prescribe different workouts almost on a weekly basis and, although this amount of variety can help to keep riders with a low attention span interested, it does very little for ticking the key training box of consistency. By repeating the same session for a number of weeks, you have a benchmark to ride to and hopefully improve on. Whether it's an average power number, cadence mark or getting a certain distance up a climb, you'll get constant feedback on your progress and real motivation to push just a bit harder.

Week 4 sees the first recovery week, during which the legs are kept spinning but are lightly loaded with high cadence workouts. Rather than a long endurance ride, some fun is prescribed with a mountain bike ride. It's important to refresh the mind as much as the body. You're then into another 3 weeks of build, leaving off where you finished at the end of Week 3. If it's going to plan, you should see a noticeable kick-up in your performance in the first strength intervals session of Week 5.

After your second recovery week of the training block, the first priority of Week 9 is retesting your FT. You drop some volume initially from your endurance ride but,

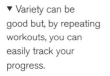
▼ Variety can be good but, by repeating workouts, you can easily track your progress.

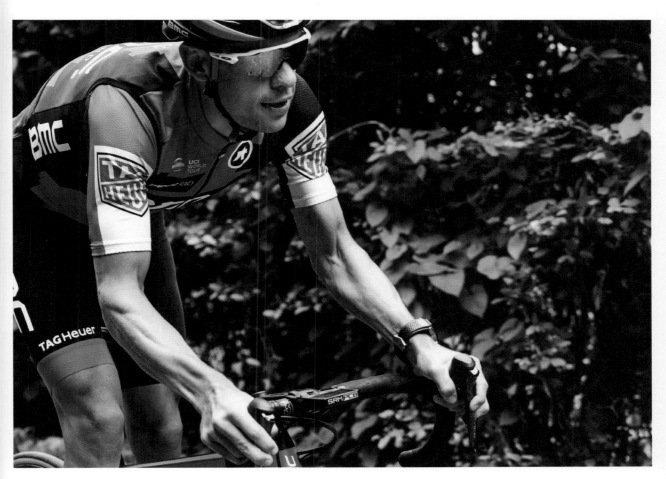

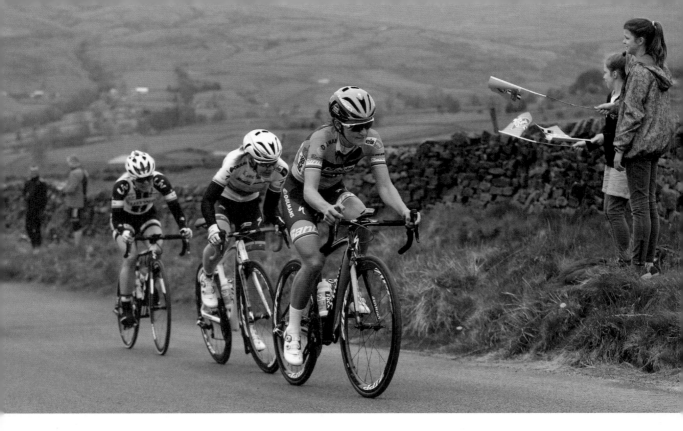

by adding in some tempo efforts, you add training load by increasing intensity. It wouldn't be a bad thing to continue through to the end of the block with two Strength Intervals sessions per week but, for the sake of sanity and to get your legs turning over a bit faster, working on 2 × 20-minute sweet spot intervals is a good choice. By the end of Week 11, you're back up to 5 hours for your endurance ride but with the tempo efforts. By the end of Week 12, your final recovery week of the block, you should have recovered from the previous three weeks, be thinking about your next block and have made significant gains.

If the block takes you up to a major target event and you want to hit your best possible form, you'd probably want to start tapering down in Week 11 rather than continuing to build. This wouldn't be as dramatic a cut in training as a recovery week but wouldn't have the volume or intensity of a build week. We'll discuss tapering further later in the chapter.

'Even for pro cyclists there's definitely been a shift in mindset from quantity to quality. I come from Australia where we've been using sports science for a while and fortunately have never had to suffer under old school high volume training plans. Our training sessions mimic our races so, although only 3–4 hours long, they always contain efforts and deliver a fair amount of intensity.' **TIFFANY CROMWELL**, CANYON/SRAM

Planning a week

One of the most common questions that's asked about training is, how much do I need to do? Riders get intimidated by the huge volumes that pro riders do and think that if they're not also putting in massive mileage, they won't improve. However, although you might be training for a big sportive or multi-day ride, it won't be anywhere near the volume of racing that the pros do. This is why they have to put in the miles they do, to be able to soak up the sheer amount of riding that full-time bike racing involves. To give you some perspective, in 2015/16, Dutch Road Race Champion Lucinda Brand averaged 1527 kilometres per month from December through to September. For the World Tour, Jonathan Vaughters, former pro and team manager of Cannondale-Drapac, has been quoted as saying that to get within spitting distance of ever riding the Tour de France requires consistent years of riding 20,000 miles a year! Even if you're racing, your races won't come near to the length of the events that the pros do, so you don't need to try to match, or even come near to, their training. What you do need to do, though, is train smart, make sure every pedal stroke is focused and has a purpose and that you eliminate junk miles. Get out of the 'more is more' mindset; quality trumps quantity every time. A great example of this is Paul Oldham, who, despite working a full-time job and typically only training on average 7 hours per week, has consistently been one the UK's top cyclo-cross racers.

◄ Don't be intimidated by or think you have to put in the weekly training volume the pros do.

Prioritise three focused bike workouts each week – yes, just three. These sessions are sacrosanct, have to be completed exactly as prescribed and are what you plan your week around. These will typically consist of two weekday higher intensity interval type sessions, often completed on a stationary bike. However, during the season, one of these may be an evening time trial, circuit race or track league. In the off season, one of these may also be a chain-gang type session with your club. The third session, usually reserved for the weekend, is your longer endurance ride. For the vast majority of riders, if they followed this structure consistently, adjusting the sessions to their goals and time of year, they would see considerable improvement.

The reasons this structure works so well is that it firstly provides plenty of flexibility, meaning that you've got some days to juggle around when life gets in the way of your riding. Secondly, you're well rested for each workout. This means you can give them 100 per cent and the intensity and training load you can achieve isn't compromised by fatigue. By being able to give a workout more, you'll get more back from it. Thirdly, by making your training volume realistic, attainable and flexible, you're far more likely to manage it week after week, which is the key to making progress. If you're too ambitious with your training planning, scheduling a workout into every spare moment, it's a recipe for failure. All it takes is a hard spell at work, your children not sleeping well or another of life's little obstacles and you're missing sessions. It's all too easy then, once you've failed on your training plan, to fall into a negative all or nothing mindset and to let your training slip completely. It's far better to give your training some breathing room, have three must-do workouts and then, if you can fit in some more without it affecting those key sessions, just see it as a bonus. You can do more than the three sessions but, if the extra riding or activity impacts negatively on the quality of your three key sessions, you have to question what you're getting out of it.

The most important rule is to prioritise those key sessions. Make sure you have a rest day before them or, if you do schedule in some activity, that it doesn't leave any fatigue in your legs.

Below is an example week taken from the 12-week off-season block we used when looking at planning a training block.

WEEK 7

Monday	Rest
Tuesday	Big gear/low cadence
Wednesday	Rest
Thursday	Big gear/low cadence
Friday	Gym/rest
Saturday	Endurance ride
Sunday	Club ride

It might seem odd to start the week with a rest day but, chances are, you will have put in at least one big ride over the weekend and need to be recovered before the demanding session planned for Tuesday. Obviously if you've done your endurance ride on the Saturday and rested on the Sunday, you could do your intervals on Monday. Wednesday is another rest day. This doesn't have to be complete inactivity (see 'Recovery weeks' below for suitable activities for rest days). Thursday is your second key interval session. On the Friday, you might choose to rest or, as many riders do throughout the off season, do some strength work in the gym. Although you've got a long ride ahead of you on the Saturday, the intensity isn't high so a degree of fatigue or stiffness in your legs isn't a problem. Towards the end of this example 12-week block, some higher intensity efforts are added to the endurance ride. As you transition into pre-season and season, the intensity of these efforts will increase. If you find that your ability to complete these efforts is compromised by your Friday session, you'll have to rethink it. The weekend is when most of us have the time to get some miles in but avoid the temptation to bury yourself and ruin the quality of the following week's training. If you are able to get out on both days, prioritise your key training ride and get that done on the Saturday. See a second weekend ride as a bonus, head out with your club or hit the trails on your mountain bike, secure in the knowledge that you've nailed another solid week of training.

Most riders are limited to the constraints of a working week and the weekends are the only real option for longer rides. Pro cyclists will tend to follow a different structure, often working in 3-day 'mini-blocks'. On Day 1, they'll do their most demanding session, often a long ride that includes some hard efforts to mimic the demands of a race. Day 2 will be shorter, interval based and fairly intense. Day 3 will be a long but fairly low-intensity endurance-style ride. They'll rest up on the fourth day but this will often involve a very light recovery ride and then they'll begin the cycle again. Some days may also be split with either two rides or with one session devoted to off the bike conditioning. If you're not normally constrained to a traditional working week or are heading to a training camp, you could try this type of structure. However, remember, when the pros aren't riding, they're resting, not having to go to work, pick the kids up from school or mow the lawn.

Recovery weeks

We've already discussed the importance of scheduling in regular recovery weeks as it's during these weeks of reduced training load that your body adapts and you become stronger. You'll still do some riding during a recovery week but the focus will be on easier, low load workouts, restorative cross training activities such as mobilisation work, yoga or Pilates (see Chapter 5) and some stress-free, enjoyable and social riding. Suitable midweek workouts include recovery ride, pre-event ride and high cadence (see Chapter 4). For your longer weekend ride, you should either perform a low volume endurance ride (approximately 50 per cent of the length of your last build-week long ride) or simply head out for an easy club/social ride or do something a bit different, such as hitting the trails on your mountain bike.

RECOVERY WEEK

Monday	Rest
Tuesday	Recovery ride
Wednesday	Rest
Thursday	High cadence
Friday	Restorative cross training/rest
Saturday	Rest
Sunday	Endurance ride 50% volume of last weekend's long ride or 'fun/social' ride/MTB

Planning a day

Where you fit your training into a day is more than likely to be governed by non-cycling demands on your time. During the week, this will often mean getting out on the bike or onto your indoor trainer after work. Think about timing your eating so you have the energy for the session (see Chapter 6) and, as much as possible, have everything set up and ready to go with minimum time wasted or will power sapping procrastination. Getting up early to fit in a session can seem like a solution but if you choose to try this, carefully monitor your tiredness levels and the quality of your workouts. Also, without any breakfast inside you, as you won't have time to digest it, you'll be limited to lower-intensity workouts.

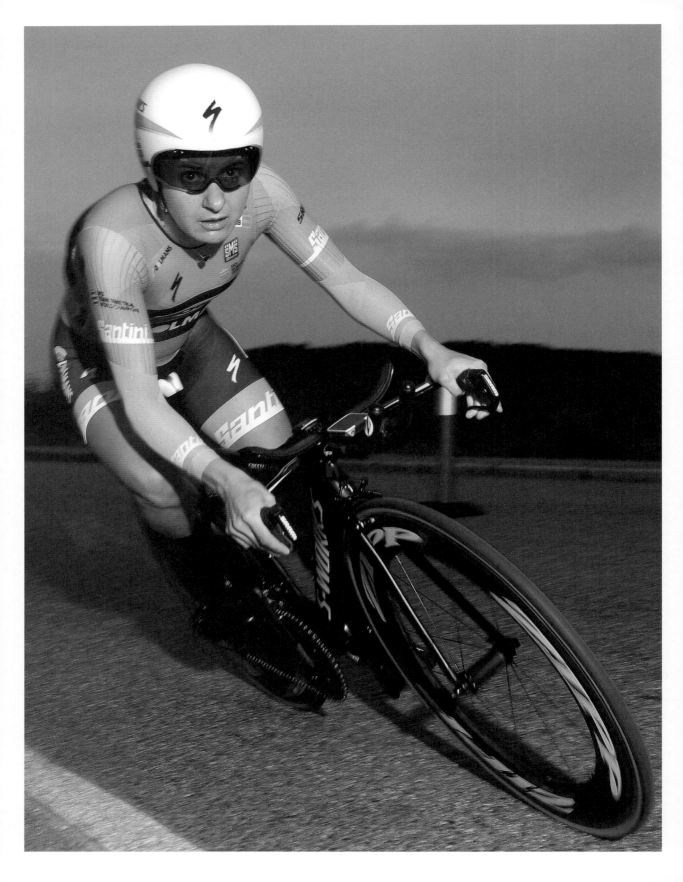

Many riders balancing cycling with a full-time job find that commuting is a time effective way to get their training in. A really good approach is to use the morning commute as an easy paced recovery ride or as a carbohydrate-fasted ride (see Chapter 4) and then, on two of your rides home, to do your interval efforts. It's fairly straightforward to find a suitable hill or stretch of road and to adapt the interval workouts to it. If you do try this approach, it's essential that on the other evenings you ride at strict recovery pace. Getting sucked into commuter racing or trying to beat your PB every night will just be junk miles, building unnecessary fatigue and reducing the quality and effectiveness of your key workouts.

Commuting, if you do it both ways, effectively means you're training split days (i.e. training twice per day). Even if you don't commute, this can be an option but, as ever, ask why you're doing it, is it benefitting you and is it impacting on your key sessions? I'm a big fan of split days, when I'll do 45–60 minutes of carbohydrate-fasted riding before breakfast and then a more intense interval session or gym work in the evening. I find I get a good physiological benefit from the morning ride, developing my fat burning ability and riding economy, and getting out first thing sets me up for the day and lifts my mood. However, because it's strictly low intensity, the training load is very low and it doesn't affect my evening session.

At the weekend, although the temptation can be to have a bit of a lie in, my advice is to get up and get the ride done. If you put it off for the sake of an extra hour in bed or waiting for a weather window, you can guarantee that something will come up and you'll end up having to cut it short or even abandon it completely. It's hard in winter, when it's cold and dark, but bed to shed or snore to door is the tough bit. Ninety-nine per cent of the time, once you're out and riding it's fine. Get all your kit ready the night before to reduce excuse-forming hurdles and ideally arrange to meet a friend to ride with.

Tapering

During a training block, you use build weeks to develop fitness and recovery weeks to allow for adaptation to this overload stimulus to occur. It's not unusual, during the final week of a 3-week build, to start to see your performance or form drop off as you'll have accumulated significant fatigue. If you're using TrainingPeaks and their Performance Management Chart, you'll be able to track this process. As you head into a target event, you'll want to minimise fatigue and, in doing so, maximise form and event day performance. Unfortunately, if you simply stopped training and rested up completely, your fatigue would drop but so would your fitness. The solution is a progressive reduction in training, which reduces fatigue, maintains fitness and maximises form. This progressive reduction in training is known as tapering. Although power meter data and analysis tools such as the Performance Management Chart allow for tapers to be planned and predicted more accurately, like all aspects of performance, we all respond differently.

In general, you should look to end your final build week 14 days before an event that you wish to peak for. Your event will probably be on a weekend, so your final

◄ To reap the rewards of your training, you have to back off and reduce your levels of fatigue, this process is tapering.

endurance focused ride would be on the Saturday or Sunday 2 weeks before your event. During the following week, you can still afford to work fairly hard during your midweek sessions but would be better focusing more on higher intensity work rather than longer intervals. Minute on/minute off (see Chapter 4) sessions would work well. For your longer weekend ride, you should be looking to cut volume by approximately 50 per cent, so if your final long ride the weekend before was 4 hours, head out for just a couple of steady Zone 2 hours this weekend. You don't want to be putting in any significant efforts but some sprints thrown into the final hour can help keep your legs feeling fresh. Any cross training activity should be fairly gentle and restorative; maybe even consider dedicating the time to getting a massage. Definitely avoid any heavy strength training and anything else that would add unnecessary fatigue to your legs. Any bonus or additional rides you've been doing on top of your three core rides should be cut completely this week.

TWO WEEKS BEFORE A BIG EVENT

Monday	Rest (following final long ride)
Tuesday	Minute on/minute off
Wednesday	Rest
Thursday	Minute on/minute off
Friday	Rest
Saturday	Restorative cross training, rest or massage
Sunday	Endurance Ride 50% volume of last weekend's long ride. Predominately Zone 2 but can include some short sprints in final hour

The week leading into your event should largely resemble a recovery week but will include a pre-event ride on the day before your event.

PRE-EVENT WEEK

Monday	Rest
Tuesday	High cadence or pre-event
Wednesday	Rest
Thursday	High cadence or pre-event
Friday	Rest
Saturday	Pre-event
Sunday	Event

It's perfectly normal during a taper to feel sluggish, tired or even slightly depressed. The reason for this is that you're not getting the hormonal high you normally get from your hard workouts and are literally going cold turkey. Stick with it, though, have faith in the weeks of consistent training you have done and don't be tempted to 'panic train' with any additional workouts. At this stage, you're not going to gain

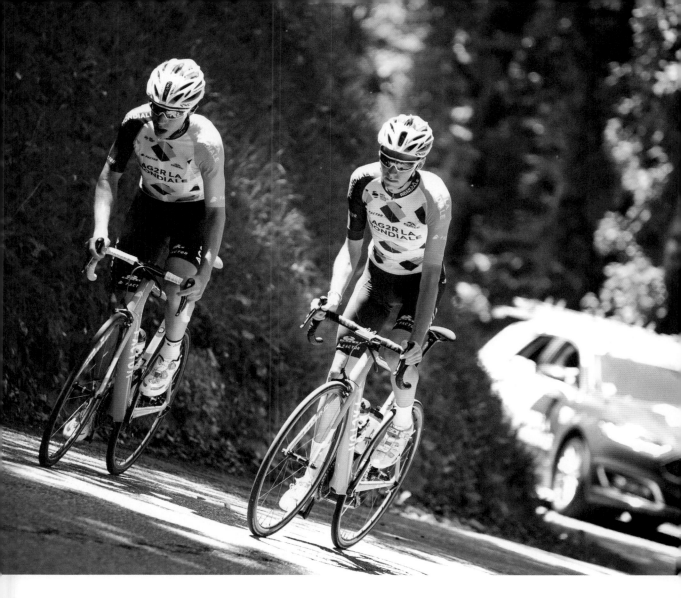

▲ Hitting your targets in a big event can be extremely motivating but you'll still need to recover before getting back into full training.

anything from additional training, you'll just add unnecessary fatigue. Take advantage of the additional time you'll have during a taper to ensure that your bike is running perfectly, all your kit and nutritional requirements are sorted and that your logistics for your event, such as travel and accommodation, are all finalised.

The week following a big event, especially if you've pushed really hard, should be a full recovery week. You might want to head out for a recovery ride (see Chapter 4) on the Monday but ensure you're extremely disciplined about keeping the intensity really low. If your event has gone really well, you may well feel super buoyed up, motivated and wanting to crack on with hard training. Avoid giving in to these euphoric feelings as, although your mind may be telling you to push on, you're likely to be extremely physically depleted and in need of full recovery.

Multiple events

Tapering fully for an event effectively rules out structured progressive training for at least 3 weeks, 2 weeks of taper and 1 week of recovery, so is a big commitment. We've previously discussed how, in an Olympic year, the Great Britain Cycling Team wouldn't go through a full taper prior to the Track Cycling World Championships. They'd train through, banking the extra training, accepting a reduced performance at the Worlds but reaping the rewards later at the Olympics.

If you're wanting to ride a number of events during the year, it's probably not realistic to follow a full taper for each one. Commit to a couple of full tapers for your 'A' events, but for less important events, 'B' priority, a mini taper of 1 week, following the pre-event week structure, would be more appropriate. You would still probably push yourself hard for a 'B' priority event and it would therefore be advisable to take a recovery week afterwards.

'C' priority events are effectively 'training events', being ridden in place of your regular long weekend ride. You wouldn't taper at all for these; you would incorporate them into build weeks but wouldn't expect a stellar performance. The ideal would be to schedule a 'C' event at the end of a 3-week build so that it was followed by a recovery week but, as long as you fuel, hydrate and pace well and don't go too deep, one could be ridden mid build. As with all aspects of performance, recovery rates and the ability to bounce back from hard rides vary massively from one rider to another. Follow the advice in Chapter 7 to optimise your recovery and experiment to find how well you recover but remember, if riding a 'C' event compromises the quality of your training for the following week, was it really worth doing?

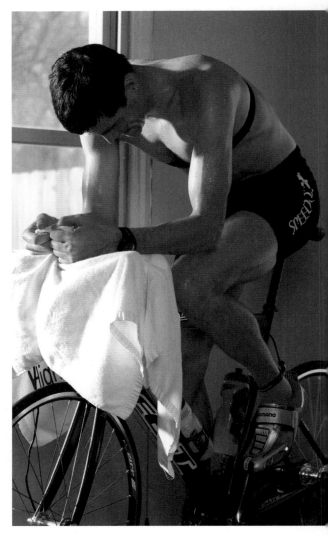

▲ Continuously hammering yourself and packing in multiple events isn't training smart and will just result in exhaustion.

Weekly racing

If you're competing in weekly racing, such as your club 10-mile time trials, track league, local criterium/crit or cyclo-cross, you obviously can't taper down every week. Again, there will be a certain amount of personal experimentation to find what works best for you, but try the following guidelines.

- All these weekly types of event tend to be of fairly short duration and, although high in intensity, the training stress they'll develop won't be too different from a hard midweek workout. The simplest approach, therefore, is to substitute it for one of your midweek sessions.
- Schedule your week to allow for a recovery day afterwards, maybe with a recovery ride, and an easy day beforehand, with a pre-event ride or high-cadence session (see Chapter 4 for specific sessions).
- Allow as much time as possible between your second midweek workout and your race.
- Consider dropping the duration of your weekend endurance ride for the 'race season'. You should already have developed a solid endurance base during the off and pre-season and can afford to just maintain this.
- Continue to work on the basis of 3 build weeks followed by a recovery week. If you find your race performance improves significantly during the recovery week or during the week following it, consider backing off your build week training and allowing more recovery during each week.
- Racing every week is a balancing act between performing at your best and keeping up training to at least maintain your fitness level. If you're committing to a period of racing, such as a two-month-long track league, you have to make a decision. Either race performance is your priority and you'll sacrifice some training gains during that period or you'll accept not performing to your peak every week and continue building fitness.

EXAMPLE BUILD WEEK WITH WEEKLY MIDWEEK EVENING EVENT

Monday	Pre-event
Tuesday	Track league, crit or TT
Wednesday	Rest/recovery ride
Thursday	Midweek workout
Friday	Gym/rest
Saturday	Endurance ride (reduced volume)
Sunday	Rest

EXAMPLE BUILD WEEK WITH WEEKLY WEEKEND EVENT

Monday	Rest/recovery ride
Tuesday	Midweek workout
Wednesday	Gym/rest
Thursday	Endurance ride (reduced volume)
Friday	Rest
Saturday	Pre-event
Sunday	Cyclo-cross race

PRO TRAINING DIARIES

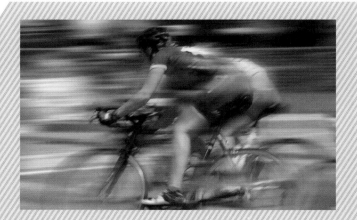

Below are three real excerpts for the training plans of riders on the Canyon/SRAM team. They're taken from the team's training camp in Majorca, from Lisa Brennauer's off season and from Barbara Guarischi's season.

TEAM TRAINING CAMP SCHEDULE, MAJORCA, DECEMBER 2016

This was the first opportunity the team had to all get together at the start of the off season. The main thing to take from this excerpt is that, even though it's very early in the off season, there's still some intensity with 'Medio" efforts, sprints and race pace work behind the car. Also, that every ride has focus and structure to it. The 3 days on followed by a rest day is fairly standard for pros who aren't constrained by the working week and, if you get the chance to go on a training camp, is definitely worth trying.

	Duration	Intensity	Content
Tuesday	n/a	n/a	Travel/Arrival
Wednesday	4 hours	Base and Medio	2 x climbs (Puig Randa): 5 x (2:30 mins @ Medio 30 secs hard acceleration seated), 4 x (2 mins @ higher Medio, 1min easy), 15 mins between sets, last 45 mins behind car, focus on higher cadence
Thursday	5 hours	Base and Medio	After 1 hour, 3 hours and 4 hours, 20 mins behind car and 4 x sprints on signal from car (3 mins easy between sprints), focus on higher speed and cadence behind car
Friday	4.5 hours	Base and Medio	After 45 mins and 3 hours, 10 mins echelon, end with a full lead out and sprint. Not echelons behind car!!!
Saturday	n/a	n/a	Rest
Sunday	4 hours	Base and Medio	2 x climbs (Puig Randa): 5x (2:30 mins @ Medio, 30 secs hard acceleration seated), 4 x (2 mins @ higher Medio, 1min easy), 15 mins between sets, last 45 mins behind car, focus on higher cadence, 4 x sprints on signal from car
Monday	5 hours	Base	Climbing day, on way home 1 x 10–15 mins echelon (without car), last hour behind car

*Medio is a zone description used by team physiologist Andreas Lang. It covers up to FTP and equates to sweet spot and lower Zone 4.

LISA BRENNAUER, OFF SEASON, JANUARY 2017

Again, despite it being the off season, there's plenty of intensity scheduled in and it's definitely not just a case of Lisa grinding out long and slow kilometres. There are two pure 'Base Rides' but even these have some focus/aims and follow either one or two harder days (see chart opposite top).

	Duration	Intensity	Content
Tuesday	4 hours	Base and Medio	After 45 mins, 1.5 hours and 2 hours 15 mins, 3 x (3 mins @ >260W, 2 mins easy). In last hour do 4 x full sprints, 5–10 mins rest between
Wednesday	n/a	n/a	Rest
Thursday	3.5 hours	Base and Anaerobic	2 x 8 mins (40 secs @ >350W, 20 secs easy), 15 mins rest. In last hour 10 mins @ >220W on flat road
Friday	4 hours	Base and Medio	2 x climbs: 1st climb: 4 x (2 mins @ Medio with 1 min easy between). 2nd climb: 10 mins @ high cadence
Saturday	5 hours	Base	Base ride, all climbs easy
Sunday	n/a	n/a	Rest
Monday	3.5 hours	Base and FTP	1 x climb: 4–5 x (2 mins @ >290W, 1 min easy). After 2–2.5h 2 x10 mins @ >230W @ higher cadence
Tuesday	4 hours	Base	Base ride, fluent and higher cadence in last hour (flat terrain)
Wednesday	Rest	Rest	

BARBARA GUARISCHI, IN SEASON

With a tough race starting this training block, it's no surprise to see Barbara taking a couple of days off the bike. She might have only had one rest day planned but it's important to listen to your body, especially after a big event, and be flexible with your training. With another race at the end of the block, it's no surprise that the training load is fairly light and, for in-season training, it's more about maintenance of form and management of fatigue rather than trying to build fitness. There's a bit of intensity, motor paced work, short 'Medio' efforts and some sprints. These are important to maintain race form.

	Duration	Intensity	Content
Sunday		Race	Ronde van Drenthe
Monday	n/a	n/a	Rest
Tuesday	n/a	n/a	Rest
Wednesday	Gym/3 hours ride	Base	Gym with focus on max strength/explosively/base ride in afternoon
Thursday	4 hours	Base	Base ride, in last 1.5–2 hours motor paced training
Friday	n/a	n/a	Rest
Saturday	4 hours	Base and Medio	After 1 hour, 2 hours, 3 hours on flat or undulating profile (4 x 2 mins @ Medio with 2 mins easy)
Sunday	3 hours	Base and sprint	After 1 hour, every 30 mins 1 x full sprint
Monday	n/a	n/a	Rest
Tuesday	n/a	n/a	Rest
Wednesday		Race	Dwars Door Vlanderen

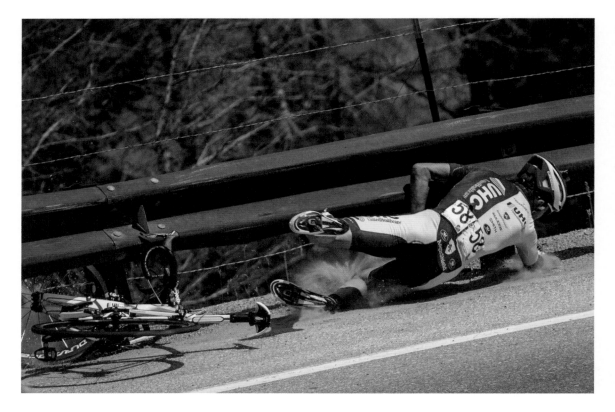

When it goes wrong

No matter how well you plan your training, illness, work or other factors often mean that you just don't manage to stick to your plan. This is one of the main reasons for making a rough year plan based around key events but only planning 8–12-week blocks in detail.

If you find you are consistently struggling to do the sessions you've planned, it's likely you've been overly ambitious and need to dial back the demands you're placing on yourself.

The odd missed session here and there is no big deal but if you miss two of your key sessions in a week, you should repeat that week. If you miss all three key sessions, go back and repeat the previous week.

If you lose more than a week of training, restart your training block at the last recovery week that you successfully completed. For example, if you were working through the 12-week block that we've been looking at, completed Week 6 but then got ill and were off your bike for two weeks, you should go back and restart the block with Week 4. The recovery week will be a relatively gentle reintroduction to structured training and, by going back, you'll take into account lost fitness and be able to rebuild it.

▲ Whether it's illness, injury, work, family or just having a bad day, things will go wrong and impact your cycling. Your training has to be adaptive to this.

For more than a few weeks of lost training, you'd probably be looking to restart the whole training block.

Obviously, if you're planning a training block towards a key event on a set date, losing or repeating weeks is a problem. The solution to this is to give yourself a 'buffer block'. If your planned block towards an event is 12 weeks, schedule it to start 16 weeks out from the event. If it all goes without a hitch, simply repeat the final 4 weeks of your block, remembering that you'll probably be following a 2-week taper. If you do lose some time, hopefully your buffer will mean that you're still in the shape you want to be for your event.

Avoiding and recovering from injury

'I tore my posterior cruciate ligament in December 2015, so not ideal with the Olympics the following year. I wasn't coached by the team coach anymore but was handed over to be put through a rehab process initially by the team doctor and then the physiotherapist and physiologist. It'd be initially injury-specific rehab exercises, it was fairly slow progress and, for a couple of weeks at least, it was just a case of practising walking. I wasn't allowed outside on a bike for two months. It was the physiologists and physiotherapist's jobs to be inventive and creative with finding ways we could cheat the recovery. That included things like single-legged turbo sessions with a weight on one side of the crank and altitude chamber work where I can stress my cardiovascular system with low power loads. I had to push but also be sensible and honest about where I was. I guess there was some luck involved but it worked.' KATIE ARCHIBALD, GREAT BRITAIN CYCLING TEAM

When it comes to developing chronic overuse injuries, cycling, compared with impact sports such as running, has an extremely low incidence rate. In fact, as such a joint-friendly activity, it's frequently prescribed for rehabilitation. Most forms of pain and discomfort on the bike (hand, wrist, neck, knee and lower back pain being the most common) can usually be corrected by a proper bike fit, remedial exercises or, most commonly, a combination of the two. The most important thing, if you do suffer from any unusual pain or discomfort on the bike, is to immediately seek qualified professional advice, a physiotherapist led bike fit being your best option. Don't just ignore pain and think it'll go away, and don't just seek the advice of clubmates or internet forums. You'll waste time trying a number of supposed cures, randomly fiddling with your bike set-up, losing quality riding time and potentially making the issue worse. An experienced physiotherapist will be able to identify the problem by taking a detailed history, conducting a physical examination and looking at your position on the bike. Without a doubt, this will be the most time efficient and effective route back to pain free cycling.

Acute injuries in cycling are usually the result of crashes and, if you choose to race, are almost inevitable. At the less severe (but still painful) end of the spectrum is

'The annual team training camp in December is really important as it's pretty much the only time of year that the whole team is together. Because of the races we do, it's only normally six riders at them and some of the support team. At camp, everyone is there. At my first Canyon SRAM camp in December 2015 I was in a cast and on crutches. I asked the team management if it was still okay for me to come out for a couple of days but they insisted on me coming out for the whole 12-day camp. This meant I could meet the team and really get to know them, which is essential if you're going to be spending half the year on the road with them trying to win bike races.' **HANNAH BARNES**, CANYON/SRAM

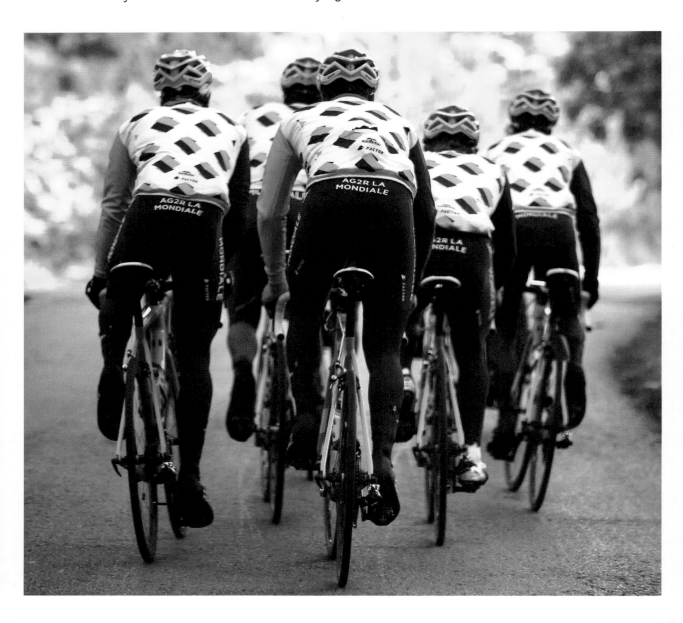

road rash. Basically a burn caused by heat generated from friction when sliding along the road or track, the priority when treating it is cleaning the wound. This can be extremely painful, especially if grit is embedded, and, for bad cases, doctors on pro teams will often administer a local anaesthetic for the cleaning process. It's usually a case of just gritting your teeth though and using a slightly abrasive sponge in the shower. Once clean, let the air get to it as much as possible but, during the night or if wearing clothes, apply a non-adhesive dressing to avoid the wound sticking to fabric. For more serious injuries, such as a broken collarbone, again the priority is getting a professional diagnosis, treatment and rehabilitation plan that you're confident in.

Some pro stories of recovery from injures are simply staggering. In the women's road race at the 2016 Rio Olympics, Dutch rider Annemiek van Vleuten, while leading the race, suffered a horrendous crash which resulted in facial injuries, severe concussion and three lumbar spinal fractures. However, in just ten days she was back on the bike, won the Lotto Belisol Belgium Tour a month later and then, in 2017, took the rainbow jersey in the time trial. Although inspirational, it's important to remember that it's a pro cyclist's job to recover fast, they'll have the very best medical care and it'll be their only focus. If you are unfortunate enough to suffer a serious injury, whether from cycling or not, that keeps you off the bike, don't rush your recovery but do seek out and follow the professional advice and support that will ensure as quick a return as possible. Consult with your doctor and physiotherapist and, in the same way as you'd produce a training plan, make a structured rehabilitation plan with key goals along the way to your full recovery.

◄ Getting a professional diagnosis that you trust and believe in is the key to a successful return from injury.

I speak from experience as, in the summer of 2015, I ruptured my patella tendon and, with a month in plaster, another two in a brace and then a further month working on getting my leg to bend again, was off my bike for over four months. I was lucky enough to be guided through my rehabilitation by former Great Britain Cycling Team physiotherapist Phil Burt, and having the confidence in his expertise and the plan we put together, was key to my successful recovery. It definitely worked and I was back on a bike in November, training properly in January and went on to win gold in the team pursuit at the World Masters track cycling championships in October 2016.

Training camps

Many riders take some time off, especially during the winter months, and head for a warm weather training camp. For pro riders, their main team training camp takes place fairly early in the off season and is a chance for testing, bike fitting, season planning and getting to know any new teammates and support staff. The actual training, while not quite secondary to these other goals, is often fairly relaxed and social.

If you're lucky enough to be able to take some time out and go on a training camp, it's an opportunity not just to get some decent riding in but, because you won't have the demands of work and family life, you'll be able to complement the riding with optimum professional-quality recovery.

There are so many great locations for a training camp. Look for a location that offers both flat and hilly rides, has good roads and, most importantly, a stable and pleasant climate. You don't need palatial accommodation but you want somewhere where you're happy chilling out when you're not riding and where you can source nutritious meals. It's also handy to have a decent bike shop nearby for spares and dealing with any mechanical issues.

'It's essential to pick somewhere with a mild climate so you don't have to go out in the rain or snow. Nutrition is key to staying healthy on a training camp. You've got the double stress of training and travel so your body needs all the nutritional support it can get. As well as fuelling your training and recovery with the macronutrients, carbohydrates, protein and fat, the micronutrients, vitamins and minerals are also really important. So, you can't just eat bread, pasta and meat, fruit and vegetables are essential.'

JULIA SCHULZE, TEAM DOCTOR, CANYON/SRAM

Because you'll have more time to devote to recovery on the camp, you can afford to push the volume of your training. We talked earlier about the 3 days on and 1 day off structure that many pros use, and this can work really well. Do your longest ride with the hardest efforts on the first day of 3, back off the duration/intensity a bit on day 2 and then, on day 3, you can still get out for a decent ride but keep the intensity low. On your mid-camp day off, you could go out for a light recovery ride but you'd probably gain more from just relaxing by the pool. Repeat the cycle for the next 3 days. Avoid the temptation to just mindlessly cram in as much riding as you possibly can – quality still trumps quantity.

It's also important to be aware, especially if temperatures are significantly higher than you're used to, that you may have to adjust your pacing and training zones accordingly. Whereas you might be able to complete an endurance ride predominately in mid to high Zone 2 at home, in higher temperatures you may have to ride at the lower end of the zone. As the camp goes on you will slowly acclimatise but this takes time and, if very high temperatures are forecast, you should ride early in the day to avoid them. This adjustment of training zones due to temperature is also something to be aware of if you're competing in an event abroad.

Because of the higher volume of training you'll be putting in and the stress of travelling, it's wise to schedule in a recovery week to effectively taper you into the camp. You should also schedule in a post-camp recovery week. Fired up by the riding that they did on their camp, many riders come home and try to maintain a similar level of training. Invariably they end up getting ill and probably negating all of the benefits from the camp. The training you did on the camp would have stressed and lowered your immune system, plus, when travelling, you're exposed to unfamiliar germs and infections. A recovery week post-camp will give your immune system

▶ Training camps can be a brilliant boost for both mind and body but avoid the temptation to ramp up your training too dramatically.

a helping hand and will also maximise your adaptations to the training load you accumulated on camp.

Another reason that many pros go on a training camp is to reap the physiological benefits of altitude. There are two main reasons for doing this. The first, if the riders are going to be taking part in a race that climbs high mountains, is to acclimatise the riders to functioning at altitude. The second is to use altitude to boost their red blood cell count and, in doing so, enhance their performance. Although not nearly as effective or predictable as using the banned drug EPO or blood transfusions, this is a legal way of increasing their blood's ability to carry oxygen. In order to get the most out of their training and obtain the blood boosting effects of altitude, the riders will live and sleep high but train low. One of the most popular pro altitude training locations is Mount Teide on Tenerife. Sited at over 2000 m, the Hotel Parador definitely ticks the 'sleep high' box, but with a 35km climb from sea-level to that point, training low is easily achieved too. At the 2010 Tour de France, Sir Bradley Wiggins struggled with long high-altitude climbs and, to remedy this, coach Tim Kerrison identified Teide as the perfect location. Since then the Teide training camp has been a Team Sky pre-Tour staple and many other top teams have followed their lead. Obviously this live high/train low approach

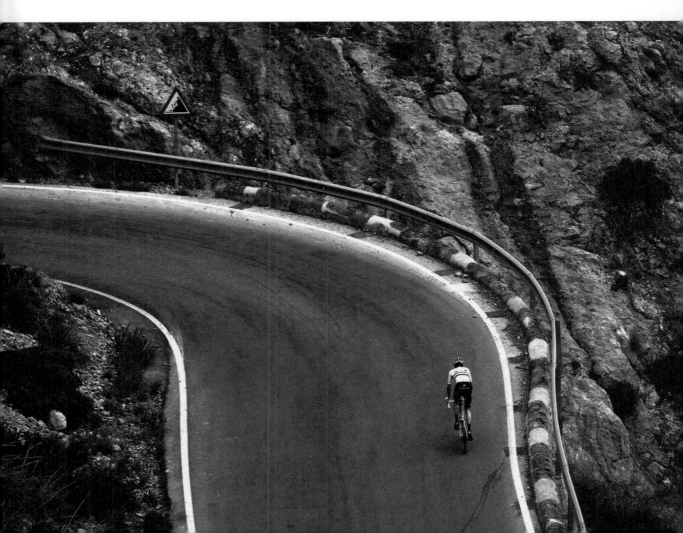

can be costly and logistically difficult, and some pros will sleep in hypoxic (low oxygen) rooms or tents in an attempt to mimic the effect of sleeping at altitude. However, like many aspects of training and performance, individual athletes' responses to altitude and the most effective protocol for them varies massively. Considerable research is still being undertaken in this area and there's no doubt that the recommendations and protocols will continue to evolve. For now, if you're considering booking time in an altitude chamber or even hiring a hypoxic tent to sleep in, there are definitely better ways to spend your money.

'Response to altitude is very much an individual thing and all the teams and riders will have their own protocols. It's really hard to do it properly though as you need to do constant blood testing and only big teams like Sky can really afford it. When I was racing in the US, for races at altitude, such as anything out of Boulder or the Tour of Gila, I knew I had to acclimatise beforehand for at least 2.5 weeks or I'd be at a big disadvantage to the locals.'

PHIL GAIMON, EX-PRO WITH GARMIN-SHARP AND CANNONDALE-DRAPAC

▼ By planning and training smart you can ensure that you leave it all on the road when it really matters.

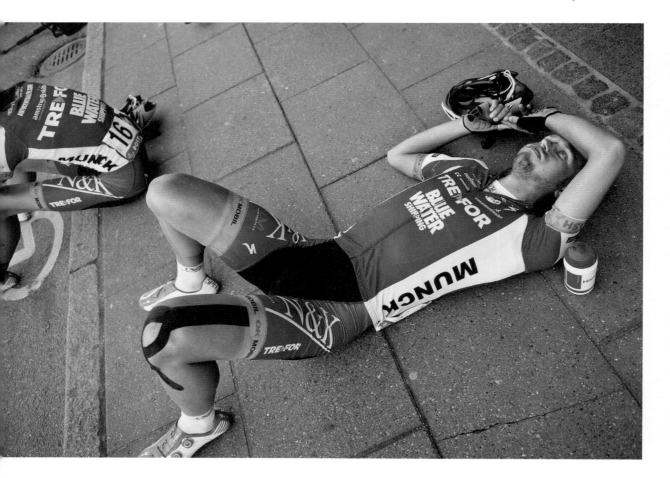

How to improve your cycling performance

Remember the fundamentals of training
When planning your training, always remember the three fundamentals of training. These are: providing your body with an overload stimulus to stimulate adaptation, progression of the training load, and the specificity of training to your sport. In addition to these fundamentals, your training has to be realistic and consistent, and must contain adequate recovery.

You're not a machine
It's vital to remember that we're all individuals and all respond differently to training. Don't mindlessly follow the same training plan as your mate and expect the same results, but listen to your body and adapt it accordingly. Monitoring training data is brilliant but don't let it dominate you and, if something doesn't feel right, it probably isn't.

Think about your event
Plan your training based on the demands of your target event and try to mimic these demands in training. If your main goal is a mountainous sportive then you'll need to put in long rides and focus on longer intervals around threshold. If you're targeting circuit races or cyclo-cross, where race durations are typically 45–60 minutes, you'll need far less volume but more intensity.

Add power to your training
A power meter doesn't just allow you to pace accurately, it provides an objective score of how stressful a session was on your body. Combined with software such as TrainingPeaks, you can track this load, see how it's affecting form, fitness and fatigue, plan tapers and even see the possible results of future training blocks. If you have some money to spend on an upgrade, forget those carbon wheels and get yourself a power meter.

Plan your year, blocks, weeks and days
Having an idea of how your riding year is going to work out, when you target events are and what training blocks you can fit in allows you to plan to train methodically. However, you shouldn't waste time planning every session in detail months ahead as, more often than not, life will throw a spanner in the works. Set goals for your training blocks and try to plan your sessions for the next 4–12 weeks. Remember to factor in non-cycling variables. You don't want a big training block to coincide with a busy time at work or to schedule in a big ride on the day of a friend's wedding, for example.

Be realistic and be flexible
When planning your training, don't pack every spare minute with workouts. A plan that is conservative but which you follow consistently will always yield better results than an overly ambitious plan followed sporadically. Remember, quality trumps quantity and recovery is as important as the workouts. By being realistic with your planning and giving yourself days off during the week and buffer weeks during training blocks, you can be more flexible and adaptable when your non-cycling life gets in the way of your riding.

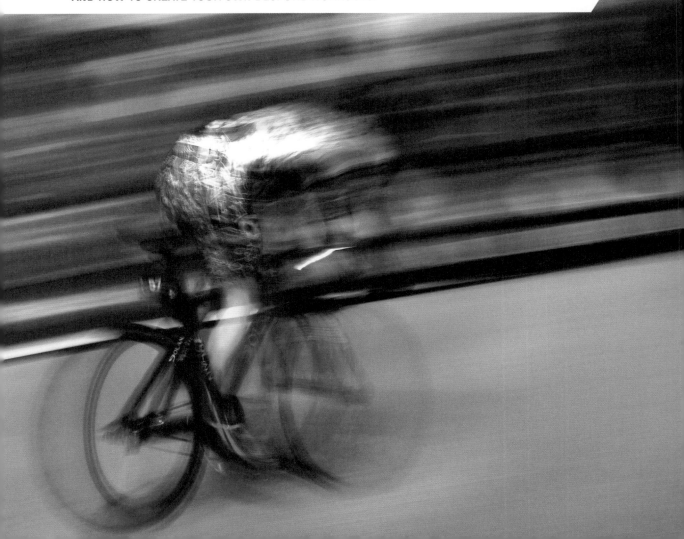

4 WORKOUT
SESSIONS AND RIDES

HAVING LEARNED HOW TO PLAN YOUR TRAINING, IN THIS CHAPTER YOU'LL FIND THE SESSIONS AND RIDES THAT WILL FORM THE CORE OF YOUR TRAINING, WHEN TO SCHEDULE THEM AND HOW TO CREATE YOUR OWN BESPOKE WORKOUTS.

'It doesn't matter if you're sprinting for an Olympic gold medal, a town sign, a trailhead, or the rest stop with the homemade brownies. If you never confront pain, you're missing the essence of the sport.' **SCOTT MARTIN**, PARALYMPIC CYCLIST

IF YOU TALK TO ANY CYCLIST, you'll find they have their favourite sessions, the workouts they dread and the ones that are the staples of their training. Most cycling magazines will have a session of the month or similar feature and there is now a massive range of video and virtual workouts. It can be confusing when faced with this plethora of choice to know which ones you should be doing and when they should fit into your training plan. Riders will often end up picking sessions almost at random, flitting between different ones or gravitating towards the workouts they enjoy the most. Unfortunately, this results in little structure to training and, in the case of the latter, usually working on existing strengths rather than addressing weaknesses.

'The sessions that really piss you off are the ones that probably do you the most good. I was just never good at sprinting, my legs don't like to go over 1000 watts so those workouts would be the ones that really hurt me and probably the ones that I most benefitted most from. The 40:20 is the nastiest workout that I used to have to do. You'll go all out for 40 seconds and you recover for 20, you do that for 10 minutes and you do 3 sets of them in a session. The 20-second recoveries get shorter and shorter and the 40s get longer and longer. That's not fun. Since I stopped racing, I'm still training, still trying to be my best at this thing, it's just I'm not doing it in a bike race anymore, but this was the one session where I told my coach I was never doing it again.'
PHIL GAIMON, EX-PRO WITH GARMIN-SHARP AND CANNONDALE-DRAPAC

The selection of workouts provided in this chapter are tried and tested sessions that should form the meat of your training plan. First of all, we discuss the importance of warming up and cooling down and the routines you should use before and after different workouts and events. Next are the midweek sessions which, although ideally suited to an indoor trainer, can also be adapted for the road. For your longer weekend rides, a base endurance ride is the standard template, but you're then given effort blocks to incorporate within it to add intensity and a guide to intervals and how to create your own workouts. Finally, we'll discuss three special rides for recovery, pre-event and carbohydrate-fasted training.

For each session, along with detailed instructions regarding training zones, cadences and durations of efforts etc, you'll also be told exactly what the session's goal is, the physiological effect it'll have, how this benefits your riding and when best to schedule it into your training plan.

◄ Chances are, the workouts you hate and avoid are probably the ones doing you the most good.

Warming up

A warm-up is essential to prepare both your mind and body for the exertion to come, whether that's a gruelling interval session, a time trial or a sportive that starts with a steep climb. Neglecting your warm-up or getting it wrong will undoubtedly compromise your performance. In training, this will mean less benefit from the session you're doing and, on event day, failing to ride to your potential.

From a physical perspective, a warm-up elicits a number of key physiological responses. It effectively switches on your aerobic system, firing up your heart and lungs and ensuring that your blood and muscles are richly oxygenated. It brings your muscles up to an optimum working temperature, allowing enzymes to function properly, energy to be delivered rapidly and for joints to move through their full range of motion. Top end and 'rev-out' type efforts in a warm-up fire up your neuromuscular system, the link between your brain and muscles, readying it for explosive and sprint efforts. A good analogy is a car starting on a cold winter's day. All of the engines parts and fuel are in place but until you've allowed the car to warm up to operating temperature, it's not going to fire effectively and efficiently when you press the accelerator and pull away.

Psychologically, a warm-up gets you in the right frame of mind for the session or race to come, focuses you and, by following a tried, tested and familiar routine, can calm you down and reduce pre-event nerves and anxiety. For midweek sessions, your warm-up serves as your transition from your working day to your workout. If you're

ALBERTO CONTADOR'S 20-MINUTE PROGRESSIVE WARM-UP

A brilliant warm-up based on the one used by Alberto Contador before time trials. Its progressive nature takes you up to threshold and then the 5-second rev-outs provide that important neuromuscular stimulus. It's suitable for both power and heart rate users and you should use your gears and/or resistance on your trainer to increase the intensity. It's also worth noting that this warm-up can be used as a short stand-alone workout if you're just wanting to turn your legs over, such as on the day before an event.

Time	Zone	Cadence	Note
0–5 mins	n/a	80–90 rpm	Very easy spinning
5–6 mins	Low Z2	90 rpm	
6–7 mins	Mid Z2	90–95 rpm	
7–8 mins	Low Z3	90–95 rpm	
8–9 mins	Mid Z3	90–95 rpm	
9–10 mins	High Z3	90–95 rpm	
10–11 mins	Mid Z4	90–95 rpm	
11–12 mins	FTP/FTHR	90–95 rpm	
12–14 mins	n/a	80–90 rpm	Very easy spinning
14–17 mins 5 secs on/55 secs off	n/a	140 rpm + 80–90 rpm	Keep resistance/gearing low for the rev-outs
17–20 mins	n/a	80–90 rpm	Very easy spinning

'Warm-ups are really important, you need to get your body ready for that effort, but my warm-up is not very long. It's 20 minutes. First, 5 minutes easy then 8 minutes progressive, so I just kick down the block every couple of minutes and then I do 2 minutes easy. Then 6-second sprints with a minute's rest in between and then recover. It's the warm-up I was taught when I was 13 by British Cycling. I love it, there's everything in that warm-up that you need.' **HANNAH BARNES**, CANYON/SRAM

on an indoor trainer, create a playlist that you always warm up to and this will then become a cue for you to forget distractions and focus on the efforts to come.

The type and length of warm-up will be determined by the nature of the session or event that follows it. A basic rule of thumb is that the shorter and more intense the main effort, the longer and more structured the warm-up will be. At one extreme of the scale are track sprinters, whose warm-up routine can sometimes be up to an hour in length. At the other end would be a minimal duration (maybe 10–15 minutes) of easy Zone 1 riding, easing into a long sportive or endurance workout. For most of the midweek workouts, you should follow either of the 20-minute warm-ups described below. This type of structure and length of warm-up is also suitable for 16km (10-mile) and 40km (25-mile) time trials, circuit races, cyclo-cross and endurance track events.

BRITISH CYCLING 20-MINUTE WARM-UP

The standard warm-up prescribed by British Cycling for all of its training plans and used by riders across the Great Britain Cycling Team. This warm-up is based on cadence so is especially suited to rollers or if you're unable to monitor heart rate or power. Both of these 20-minute warm-ups work well; it's a case of finding which suits you and the workout/event you're doing best.

I use Alberto's warm-up before time trials and pursuit efforts, and the British Cycling warm-up before indoor trainer sessions and at track league. Experiment with both and find what suits you and the particular events you're doing.

Time	Cadence	Note
0–5 mins	90 rpm	Keep resistance/ gearing low through- out the warm-up
5–7 mins	95 rpm	
7–9 mins	100 rpm	
9–11 mins	105 rpm	
11 mins–12 mins 30 secs	110 rpm	
12 mins 30 secs–13 mins	120–130 rpm	
13–15 mins	90 rpm	
15–18 mins		
6 secs on/54 secs off	150 rpm + 90 rpm	
18–20 mins	90 rpm	

TIMING YOUR WARM-UP

For workouts, the main block of the training session immediately follows the warm-up, but how should you time your warm-up when racing? The ideal is that you should start your event within 5–30 minutes of completing your warm-up. Any longer than this and you'll have effectively cooled down again. Using the example of a typical time trial, once you've signed on and got your start time,

work back from it. Aim to have your 20-minute warm-up completed 10–15 minutes before your start, giving you time for a final toilet stop and factoring in a gentle spin to the start. Many riders like to take a gel, often caffeinated, at the start of their warm-up so that it's kicking in for their race effort starting.

Some events are trickier to time, track meets being especially difficult. You'll get a schedule of races but it'll tend to be just a running order without timings. You have to estimate the duration of the events preceding yours but with crashes, false starts and other delays possible, you have to be adaptable. Try to time your warm-up as accurately as possible, take your cue from other racers in your group and don't stress if things don't go exactly to plan. These sorts of delays even happen at the Olympics and, for this reason, the Great Britain Cycling Team have used heated over-trousers to keep their athletes' legs warm. You don't need to go to these extremes but keep gently spinning on your rollers, put on a tracksuit or just cover your legs with a blanket or towel.

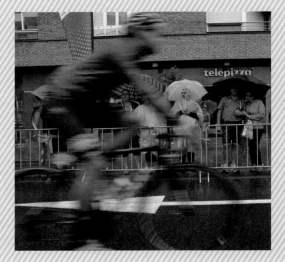

◀ Try to time your warm-up so that you're ready to go 10-15 minutes before your start time.

Warming up on the road

If you're completing the midweek workouts on the road or are competing in an event, such as a time trial, circuit race or cyclo-cross race, and don't have access to a turbo trainer, you should try to replicate one of the 20-minute warm-ups as closely as possible on a quiet stretch of road. Spend at least 5 minutes spinning easily and then build intensity progressively for 10 minutes, finishing with 1–2 minutes at FT. Recover from this effort and then aim to complete 3 × 5–6-second low gear/high cadence rev-outs with the rest of the minute as recovery. Spin easily for a couple of minutes and you're ready to go.

For your longer endurance rides, there's no need for such a progressive warm-up. Try to spin easy in Zone 1 for 10–15 minutes at the start of the ride and, if you've got some higher intensity efforts to do, try to allow yourself 20 minutes of riding before them and include a progressive build through your zones and some short rev-outs.

Cooling down

In the same way that you should progressively warm your body up in preparation for exertion, a cool-down, physically and psychologically, winds you back down. One of the innovations that Team Sky brought to the pro peloton was its riders warming down on turbos after mountaintop or sprint finishes. Although riders had traditionally ridden to their hotel as an informal cool-down, this was usually hit or miss, and often a chilling rather than progressively cooling descent. By having their turbos set up and ready to go, every rider gets exactly the cool-down they need and, although initially ridiculed by other teams, it's now the norm. It doesn't need to be as structured as a warm-up but, at the end of every ride, workout or event, you should aim to finish with at least 10 minutes of Zone 1 easy spinning. This will allow your heart rate to drop, flush metabolites out of your muscles and return your body to its resting state. Use the time to evaluate how the session you've just completed has gone and try to view the cool-down as not just the end of what you've just done, but the start of your recovery for your next ride.

▼ The cool-down at the end of your ride is as important as the warm-up at the start.

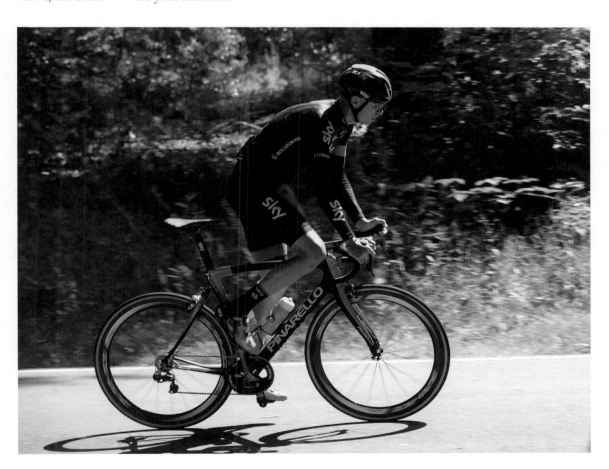

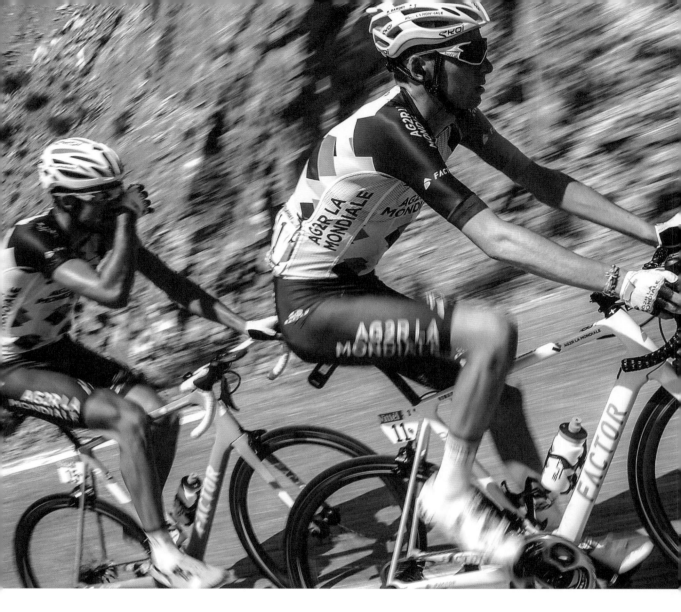

'As a sprinter, it's weird because on a sprint training day, I have to be really up for it. There's one session that I've just been given by my coach which is called Under/Overs. You do 110% FTP for 30 seconds then 95% FTP for a minute seven times through. I definitely don't enjoy it. I know it's going to really hurt so when I see that on my training I'm not thrilled. It's so hard but I know it's doing me good.'

HANNAH BARNES, CANYON/SRAM

▲ Quality is the key to effective midweek sessions. It's better to do four intervals bang on target than six sub par ones.

Midweek workouts

The following eight workouts are your midweek staples. Although designed primarily for indoor trainers, which have the main advantage of being able to control effort and intensity exactly without distraction, they can easily be adapted to road.

You'll notice that many of the sessions give you an option for the amount of reps you perform. Start with the lower figure and, as you get stronger, increase the number of reps. However, if you're not hitting the intensities required for the rep, don't just carry on. Remember, quality always trumps quantity.

STRENGTH INTERVALS

Session duration: 65–85 mins

What is it? Strength or high gear/low cadence intervals are essentially on the bike 'resistance training'.
Why? They're a highly effective way to build cycling-specific strength.
When? During the off season, as they can leave the legs feeling slow and heavy.
Notes: Despite the big gear and slow cadence, try to keep your pedal stroke smooth and avoid stamping on the pedals. Keep your upper body relaxed and your trunk still, stable and strong. Don't wrestle your bike!

Warm-up: 20 mins warm-up

Main set
5 mins
- Select a gear/resistance/hill that just allows you to hold 50–60 rpm
- Break the 5 minutes into 2 minutes seated, 1 standing and 2 seated
- Don't worry about heart rate or power zones but expect to be in Zones 4–5

5 mins Easy spinning Zone 1 recovery

Repeat for a total of 4–6 efforts (Do not do the 5-minute recovery after your final 5-minute effort, go straight into cool-down).

Cool-down: 10 mins easy spinning Zone 1

20-MINUTE INTERVALS

Session duration: 80 mins

What is it? Long 20-minute intervals that, depending on time of year and fitness level, vary in intensity from tempo (Zone 3) to threshold (Zone 4).
Why? A classic workout for raising FT and for learning to pace an extended effort.
When? A staple for the off season, pre-season and even, as a best bang for your buck workout, in season. Choose tempo in early off season, build to sweet spot and aim to be hitting threshold numbers in the pre-season. In season, back it off to sweet spot.
Notes: If I were limited to just one workout, it'd be this one and probably performed at sweet spot (mid Zone 3 – mid Zone 4) intensity. Do this twice a week, with a longer ride at the weekend, for the rest of your cycling life and, although it'd be a fairly dull existence and you'd be lacking a bit of a finishing kick, you'd still be a pretty solid rider.

Warm-up: 20 mins warm-up

Main set
20 mins
- Tempo (Zone 3), sweet spot (mid Zone 3 – mid Zone 4) or threshold (Zone 4)
- Cadence should be 90–95 rpm

10 mins Easy spinning Zone 1 recovery

Repeat for a second 20-minute effort (do not do the 10-minute recovery after your second 20-minute effort, go straight into cool-down).

Cool-down: 10 mins easy spinning Zone 1

THRESHOLD CRISS-CROSS INTERVALS

Session duration: 65–85 mins

What is it? 10-minute intervals that have you working just above and just below your FT.
Why? For boosting FT and learning to recover while still working relatively hard, essential for racing.
When? Pre-season.
Notes: This workout is so much easier to pace accurately using a power meter. It's doable for heart rate users but will require a certain amount of feel and intuition as the heart rate rise and fall will lag behind.

Warm-up: 20 mins warm-up

Main set
10 mins
• Alternating 1 min sweet spot (mid Zone 3 – mid Zone 4) with 1min low Zone 5
• Cadence should be 90–95 rpm

5 mins Easy spinning Zone 1 recovery

Repeat for a total of 2–4 efforts (do not do the 5-minute recovery after your final 10-minute effort, go straight into cool-down).

Cool-down: 10 mins easy spinning Zone 1

5-MINUTE ZONE 5 INTERVALS

Session duration: 51–67 mins

What is it? 5-minute Zone 5 VO2 efforts.
Why? Working above FT is highly effective for raising it. This intensity is also relevant for steep climbs or bridging a gap.
When? Pre-season.
Notes: If using heart rate, don't go off too hard. Your heart rate going up will lag behind the effort you're making, so build through Zones 3–4 in the first minute of each effort rather than trying to hit Zone 5 straight away.

Warm-up: 20 mins warm-up

Main set
5 mins
• Zone 5
• Cadence should be 90–95 rpm

3 mins Easy spinning Zone 1 recovery

Repeat for a total of 3–5 efforts (do not do the 3-minute recovery after your final 5-minute effort, go straight into cool-down).

Cool-down: 10 mins easy spinning Zone 1

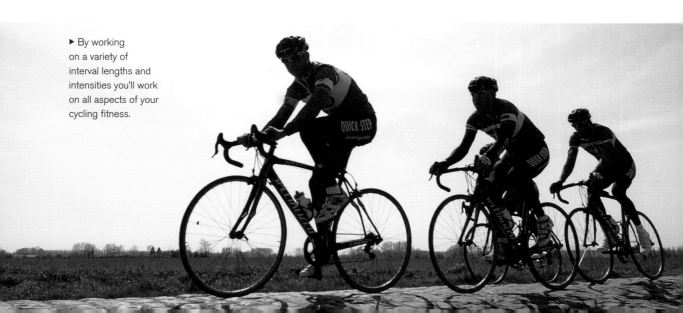

▶ By working on a variety of interval lengths and intensities you'll work on all aspects of your cycling fitness.

MINUTE ON/MINUTE OFF INTERVALS

Session duration: 55–70 mins

What is it? 1-minute Zone 6 efforts with equal length recoveries.
Why? Developing anaerobic capacity and the ability to make repeated top end efforts. Relevant to circuit, track and cyclo-cross racing.
When? In season.
Notes: Accelerate maximally at the start of the effort and then settle into a hard but sustainable output for the rest of the minute. For power users, this will be Zone 6.

Warm-up: 20 mins warm-up

Main set
10 mins
- Alternating 1 min near maximal with 1 min Zone 1 easy spinning
- Cadence at the start of the hard minute should be 100 rpm+ and then drop to a sustainable level

5 mins Easy spinning Zone 1 recovery

Repeat for a total of 2–3 efforts. (Do not do the 5-minute recovery after your final 10-minute effort, go straight into cool-down).

Cool-down: 10 mins easy spinning Zone 1

KITCHEN SINK PYRAMID INTERVALS

Session duration: 78 mins 30 seconds

What is it? As the name suggests, a mixed bag of efforts and intensities testing you from maximal sprints to sustained efforts.
Why? Race-specific session that'll sharpen your legs and prepare you for the stop-go nature of many forms of bike racing.
When? Pre-season and in season.
Notes: Make sure that the 15-second efforts are 100%. Cadence is only specified for the 5 mins efforts. Self-select for the 15 secs and 1 mins but aim for 100 rpm+

Warm-up: 20 mins warm-up

Main set
4 × 15 secs all-out, 45 secs recoveries (go straight into 5-minute recovery after final 15-second effort)

5 mins Easy spinning Zone 1 recovery

3 × 1 min Max effort Zone 6 for power users, 2 mins recoveries (go straight into 5-minute recovery after final 1-minute effort)

5 mins Easy spinning Zone 1 recovery

2 × 5 mins
- Zone 5
- Cadence 95 rpm, 3 mins recoveries (go straight into 5-minute recovery after second 5-minute effort)

5 mins Easy spinning Zone 1 recovery

2 × 1 min Max effort Zone 6 for power users, 2 mins recoveries (go straight into 5-minute recovery after second 1-minute effort)

5 mins Easy spinning Zone 1 recovery

3 × 15 secs all-out, 45 secs recoveries (go straight into cool-down after final 15-second effort)

Cool-down: 10 mins easy spinning Zone 1

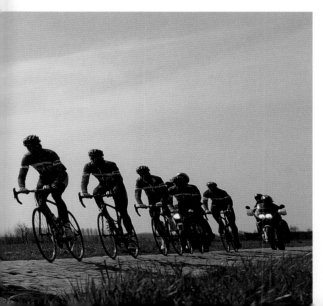

Session duration: 34–48 mins

What is it? High-intensity intervals with very short recoveries. Named after the Japanese sports scientist who first studied the effects of this type of training.
Why? Incredibly time-effective training session, proven to boost both aerobic and anaerobic capacity. Great to throw into an evening commute. Even a one rep session is worth doing and is great for fitting in a quick session when you're short of time.
When? In season.
Notes: These really hurt but make sure that the 20-second efforts are 100% even though you'll feel you're riding through treacle.

Warm-up: 20 mins warm-up

Main set
8 × 20 secs Max effort, 10 secs recovery

3 mins Easy spinning Zone 1 recovery

Complete 1–3 reps. (Do not do the 3-minute recovery after your final 4-minute Tabata block, go straight into cool-down.)

Cool-down: 10 mins easy spinning Zone 1

Session duration: 49 mins

What is it? High-cadence 'rev-out' efforts.
Why? To develop leg speed, smooth pedalling and for a relatively light leg loosening workout for recovery weeks.
When? Any time of year.
Notes: Either perform on rollers or drop gear/resistance very low. Avoid bouncing in the saddle and keep your upper body still and relaxed. Don't worry about heart rate or power zones, this session is all about cadence.

Warm-up: 20 mins warm-up

Main set
8 mins Alternating 15 secs 150 rpm + / 45 secs easy spinning

3 mins 90 rpm easy spinning

Repeat. (Do not do the 5-minute recovery after your second time through, go straight into cool-down).

Cool-down: 10 mins easy spinning Zone 1

MIDWEEK SESSIONS SUMMARY TABLE

Session name	Session duration	When to do it
Strength intervals	65–85 mins	Off season
20-minute intervals	80 mins	All year (shifting intensity)
Threshold criss-cross	65–85 mins	Pre-season
5-minute Zone 5 intervals	51–67 mins	Pre-season
Kitchen sink	78 mins 30 secs	Pre-season
Minute on/minute off intervals	55–70 mins	In season
Tabata	34–48 mins	In season
High cadence	49 mins	All year

▶ Especially if you're targeting time trials, make sure you perform interval sessions in your race position.

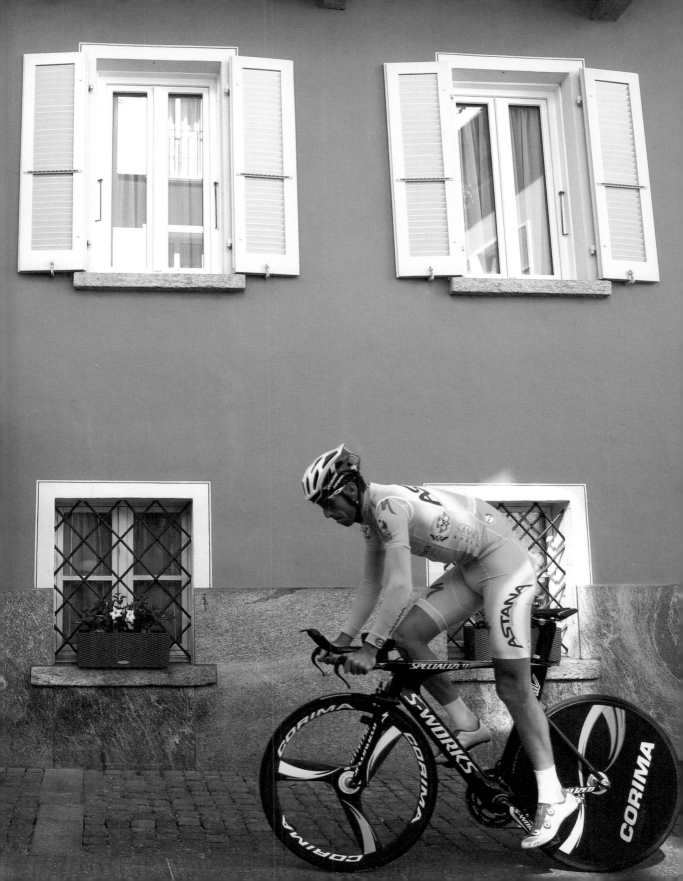

Weekend rides

For most riders, the weekend is their one chance to get out and put in some decent miles. However, without some focus and structure, it's easy to waste this precious time. These rides are your opportunity to practise your pacing, fuelling and nutrition strategies, crucial to optimising your performance on event day. Always try to have a purpose and a plan for your weekend rides rather than just heading out and accumulating junk miles.

How long does it have to be?

Think about your target events and goals. If you're aiming towards a big sportive such as the Étape or a multi-day event with long days, you should probably be aiming for 5- or even 6-hour days in the saddle. If, however, your main objectives are 16km (10-mile) or 40km (25-mile) time trials, cyclo-cross, track or circuit races, your endurance rides probably don't need to exceed the 3–4-hour mark. If you've already got a decent base, you could probably get away with just a couple of hours for endurance maintenance.

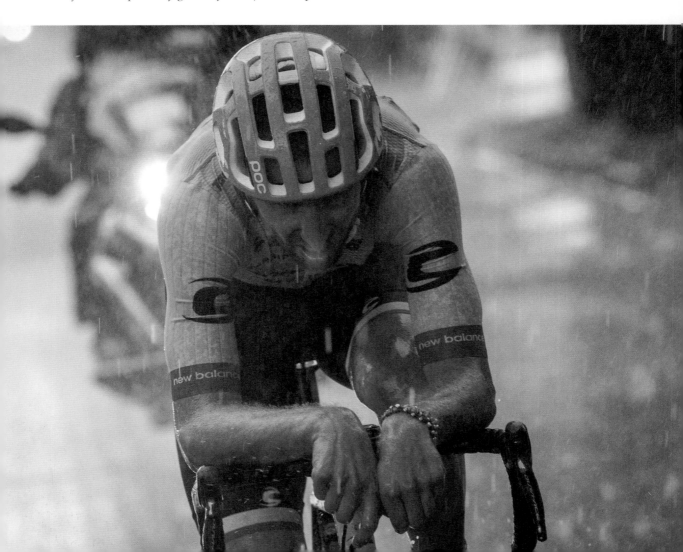

The café stop

Although a decent cup of coffee and maybe even a slice of cake can enhance the enjoyment of any ride, it does affect the benefit you'll get from it. A 4-hour ride with a 30-minute café stop in the middle is physiologically very different to a continuous 4 hours in the saddle. If you're serious about improving your endurance, either forego the café stop or schedule it towards the end of the ride. One option I use a fair bit during the winter, when a warming cup of coffee is a necessity mid-ride, is to do the first 2 hours of the ride carbohydrate-fasted (see later in chapter) to the café. I'll then have coffee and a pastry to boost warmth and blood sugar, and, continuing to feed on the way home, include some tempo or sweet spot efforts.

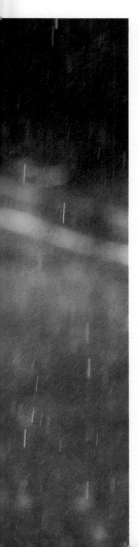

▼ Your target events will determine the length of your long ride. Don't ride for hours just for the sake of it.

Sunday club run

From a social perspective and for working on group riding skills, a club run is hard to beat but it's not the place for structured training. If you try to incorporate your own riding agenda into the club run, you'll only frustrate yourself and other riders. Last winter we had a rider who, on a few Sundays in a row, would almost grind to a halt on even the slightest incline and, as we had a 'no rider dropped' policy, we spent ages waiting for him. It turned out he was following a strict traditional base plan and didn't want to let his heart rate rise out of Zone 1.

If you want to take part in your club run, get your focused endurance ride done on the Saturday and then ride with the club on the Sunday. Sit in the wheels and take it easy; don't be tempted to contest any of the town sign sprints or attack the climbs. This is an additional ride to your core three sessions and, as such, shouldn't accumulate excessive fatigue in your legs.

Bad weather

If you're not lucky enough to live in a mild and dry climate or the pro option of migrating to Girona for the winter isn't viable for you, you're going to face and have to deal with bad weather.

With modern hi-tech clothing, you can stay amazingly comfortable in the most atrocious conditions. Layer well, invest in a decent hardshell jacket, look after your extremities (head, hands and feet) and take a good dose of toughen up. Choose flatter routes in bad weather as it'll generally be a bit warmer lower down. It's also easier to maintain a consistent intensity, and without climbs making you overly sweaty and then descents chilling you, you'll stay more comfortable.

However, whether it's snow, ice or fog, there are winter conditions when it's simply not safe to ride on the roads. Be sensible – it's better to miss one weekend ride than to risk an accident costing you weeks or months off riding, or even worse. If you live in a temperate climate, such as the UK, chances are the cold snap won't last long and the number of unrideable weekends over the course of a winter will actually be very low.

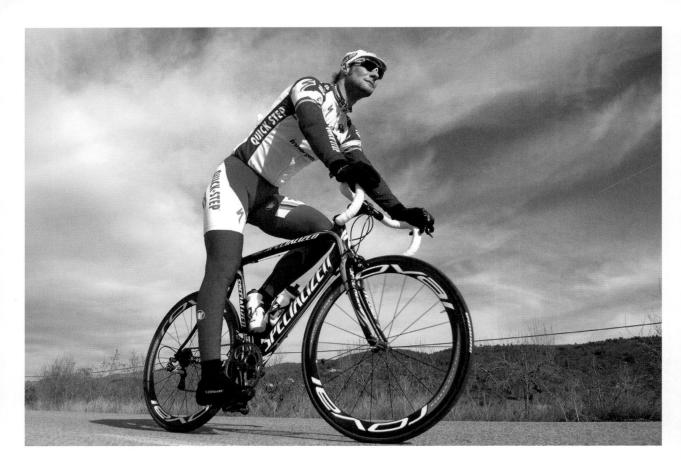

I know there are some riders, with more willpower and tolerance for boredom than I have, who will get on their indoor trainer and knock out the 3–4-hour endurance ride they originally had planned. I even had one friend, who was particularly rain averse, who would turbo through the original Star Wars trilogy! If you can manage to put in long indoor rides, brilliant, but my absolute limit is 2 hours. I'll take the view that, chances are, I'll be able to get out the next weekend and, following the quality trumping quantity mantra, will opt for some longer intervals. Twenty-minute intervals tend to be my go-to bad weather weekend workout, adjusting their intensity to the time of year. With an extra 20 minutes of Zone 2 riding either side of the intervals, it stacks up to 2 hours and without question is a decent workout. Those snowy or icy days, when the roads aren't a safe option, are when having a mountain bike or cyclo-cross bike to turn to can save your long weekend ride. You might not cover quite the same distance but you can certainly get in the saddle time, have some fun and improve your bike handling skills.

For some riders, however, especially those living in certain areas of North America, unrideable conditions can last for weeks on end. The indoor trainer can be your only option and that's when virtual reality and interactive trainers can be genuine sanity savers. You might also want to consider snow-friendly cross training activities such as 'fat-biking', snow-shoeing and cross-country skiing.

▲ For the sake of your bike handling and sanity, try to do your long rides out on the road or trails.

Weekend/longer rides

BASE ENDURANCE RIDES

Session duration: 2 hours +

What is it? Simple long, steady distance.
Why? To build endurance and to practise your pacing and fuelling strategies for longer events.
When? Throughout the year but predominately off season.
Notes: Flat or gently rolling roads make holding the solid Zone 2 effort easier.

Warm-up: 15 mins Zone 1 easy spinning

Main set
2 hours +
- As much as possible in Zone 2
- Allow to rise to Zone 3 on climbs but don't force it up

Cool-down: Final 10 mins easy spinning Zone 1

Effort blocks within endurance rides

As we've already seen, although there is a place for pure base endurance rides, especially if it's early in the off season or you're on a multi-day training camp, adding some intensity will maximise your returns from your time on the bike.

In general, you should be aiming to replicate the efforts that you're working on in your midweek workouts. In fact, you can take those sessions and slot them into your longer rides. I would recommend using the first hour of the ride to warm up and to get in some solid Zone 2 riding.

During the second, third or even fourth hours, depending on the length of the ride, include your main efforts. You'll need to plan your route to accommodate these, looking for uninterrupted stretches of road that allow you to hold your target intensity for the required duration. Follow the same effort length and recovery guidelines as specified by the relevant midweek workout and, for the rest of the time, ride solid Zone 2.

With your efforts done, make sure you allow at least 10–15 minutes of easy Zone 1 spinning to cool down. If you're wanting and able to carry on riding for more time, including some 10–20-second sprints in the final hour is great for maintaining sharpness and adding some variety. Aim to do one every 10 minutes, completing your final one with 10 minutes to go to the end of the ride. I'll always try to include these sprints, even in the last hour of a pure base endurance ride, as they always feel good and break up the monotony a bit.

EARLY OFF SEASON 3 HOURS

| First hour | **15 mins** Zone 1 easy spinning |
| | **45 mins** Solid Zone 2 |

| Second hour | **2 × 20 mins** Zone 3 Tempo (see 20-minute intervals) or |
| | **4 x 5 mins** High gear/low cadence (see strength intervals) |

| Third hour | **0–50 mins** Zone 2 with 20-sec sprint every 10 minutes |
| | **50–60 mins** Easy spinning Zone 1 cool-down |

OFF SEASON 4 HOURS

| First hour | **15 mins** Zone 1 easy spinning |
| | **45 mins** Solid Zone 2 |

| Second hour | **2 × 20 mins** Zone 3/4 sweet spot (see 20-minute intervals) |

| Third hour | **2 × 10 mins** Threshold criss-cross (see threshold criss-cross intervals) |

| Fourth hour | **0–50 mins** Zone 2 with 20-sec sprint every 10 minutes |
| | **50–60 mins** Easy spinning Zone 1 cool-down |

PRE-SEASON 3 HOURS

| First hour | **15 mins** Zone 1 easy spinning |
| | **45 mins** Solid Zone 2 |

| Second hour | **5 × 5 mins** Zone 5 VO2 efforts (see 5-minute Zone 5 intervals) |

| Third hour | **0–50 mins** Zone 2 with 20-secs sprint every 10 minutes |
| | **50–60 mins** Easy spinning Zone 1 cool-down |

IN SEASON 2 HOURS

| First hour | **20 mins** Replicate British Cycling 20-minute warm-up |
| | **20–60 mins** **2 × 10 mins** minute on/minute off (see minute on/minute off intervals) |

| Second hour | **0–50 mins** Zone 2 with 20-secs sprint every 10 minutes |
| | **50–60 mins** Easy spinning Zone 1 cool-down |

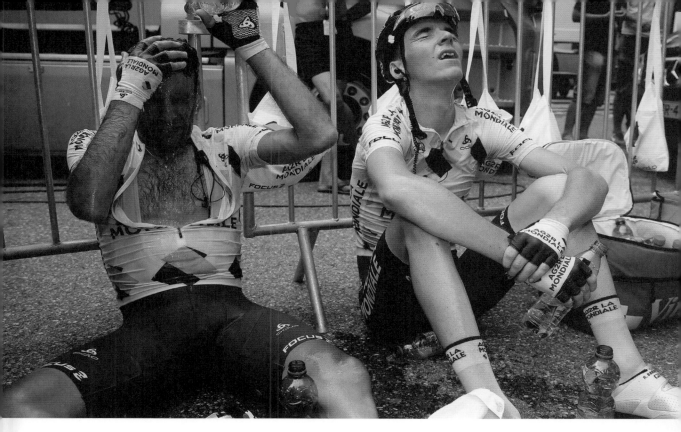

Typical effort lengths and recoveries

In addition to using the midweek workouts as a guide to effort length and recoveries to include in your endurance rides, you can also refer to the table overleaf.

Use the guidelines in the table to plan effort blocks within longer rides, to create your own midweek workouts or to add some quality work to your commutes. Simply select the zone/intensity you're looking to train, decide on an effort length and divide total effort volume by effort length to find the number of reps you'll need to do. Then follow the guidelines below to determine recovery time. Expect to have to tweak the session slightly after you've tried it but it'll be fairly near the mark.

For example, if you find the 5-minute Zone 5 intervals session too tough or daunting, even if just doing three reps, how about changing it to 5 × 3 minutes with 3-minute recoveries? The training effect will be very similar. Just add your 20-minute warm-up, a cool-down and you've got your own bespoke session. Similarly, do you dread 20-minute Intervals at Threshold? I don't blame you! I've known athletes get so worked up and psyched out by a session they dread that it dominates their entire day and they often end up skipping it. In this case, tweak the session to something more manageable, such as 4 × 10 mins with 5-minute recoveries. The total time spent at Threshold is the same and the differences in training effect would be minimal.

Zone	Title	Effort length	Total effort volume	Recovery
3	Tempo	20 mins – 2 hrs +	40 mins – 2hrs +	0–5 mins
3/4	Sweet spot	10–60 mins	40–60 mins	2–10 mins
4	Threshold	5–40 mins	40–60 mins	2–10 mins
5	VO2	2–8 mins	15–25 mins	2–5 mins
6	Anaerobic capacity + sprints	5 secs – 1 min	25 secs – 10 mins	10 secs – 15 mins +

Notes on table and specific zones

ZONE 3: TEMPO In Chapter 2 we referred to tempo as 'intensive endurance' and well-trained riders would be able to hold this intensity for long durations. It's not an intensity that you'd probably select for dedicated efforts as it's not hard enough to stimulate significant gains but does accumulate fatigue. As such, it's a bit of a physiological no-man's-land. As shown in the endurance ride examples, you might include some 20-minute Zone 3 blocks in the early off season but would be looking to step those up to sweet spot and threshold.

ZONE 3/4: SWEET SPOT Although only a subtle shift in intensity, training in upper Zone 3 and lower Zone 4 seems to have much more benefit than tempo and is great for adding intensity to your rides during the off season or for a slightly less demanding session than working at threshold any time of year. For shorter efforts at this intensity, recovery should be minimal, but a longer effort of 40 minutes, for example, might necessitate 10 minutes of easy spinning.

ZONE 4: THRESHOLD Threshold efforts can be your go-to intensity at any time of year but are classically scheduled later in the off season and into the pre-season. They're tough sessions, though, so need to be carefully used in season so as not to affect event performance. Remember, the upper end of Zone 4 is your FTP/FTHR so, in theory, this is the absolute maximum you could hold for an hour. However, the classic effort length for this intensity is 20 minutes, where you should be aiming to hold close to your FTP/FTHR. This sort of effort would require a 10-minute recovery before repeating but a session compromising multiple 5-minute threshold efforts would only require 2-minute recoveries.

ZONE 5: VO2 Zone 5 work is primarily for the pre-season and in season, although, even more so than with Threshold work, be careful not to allow demanding VO2 sessions to impact on events. As a general rule of thumb, for Zone 5 sessions, recovery length should be equal to effort length. However, if you find you're struggling to

▶ Use the sessions suggested in this chapter and the table above to create your own killer workouts and effort blocks.

maintain quality, you might have been overly ambitious and need to dial down effort length and/or rep number and also potentially up recovery.

ZONE 6: ANAEROBIC CAPACITY + SPRINTS Some 'sprint work', such as sprints within an endurance ride or low gear/resistance leg speed work, can be included throughout the year. However, dedicated sprint sessions are for pre-season and in season.

The exact nature of these top-end sessions very much depends on what you're looking to achieve from them. The 20-second sprints, which I like to include in the final hour of my endurance rides, add variety and remind your legs that cycling isn't just about grinding out steady miles. Tabata HIIT (high intensity interval training) type sessions, which schedule minimal recovery, work on your ability to sprint repeatedly and recover. Minute on/minute off type sessions develop sprint endurance. Rev-outs

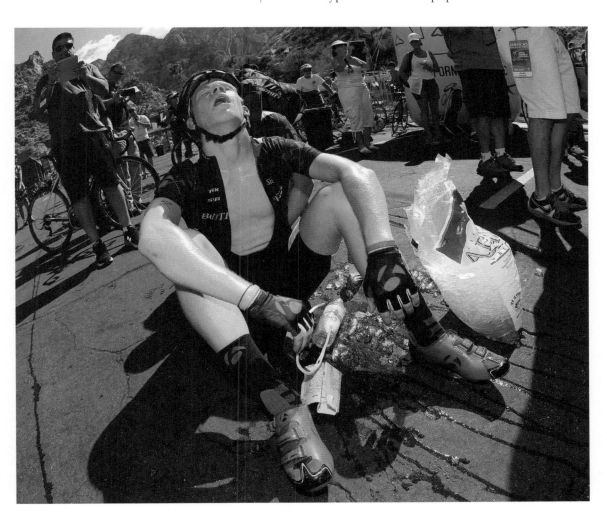

work on leg speed with low resistance. At the extreme end of quality sprint sessions, track sprinters will do as little as a 5-second maximal start effort and then recover for 15–30 minutes before repeating. Recovery is total recovery, too, usually lounging on a beanbag in the track centre, but they squeeze absolutely everything out of their muscles in that 5 seconds.

If the quality of the sprint effort is your priority, you have to ensure that recovery is adequate to allow this. However, if you're looking to build your ability to sprint, recover and sprint again, such as you'd do in a circuit, cyclo-cross or endurance track event, you're looking to not fully recover.

SMART TRAINERS AND TRAINING APPS

For midweek workouts especially, many riders now use a smart indoor trainer with an Erg mode that allows them to set wattage values for an interval and then, by adjusting the resistance to their cadence, automatically holds them at that intensity. Most of these trainers, either by using the head unit or a third party app, allow you to create such structured workouts meaning you can program

in any of the sessions described or, use the table to create your own. If you like to use an app, such as Zwift, Sufferfest, Trainerroad or others, which already have workouts, all you need to do is to either cross compare the efforts in the session to the table and determine the physiological objectives of the session or look to see what intensity or training effect the session is described as giving.

▼ Smart trainers can take the quality and effectiveness of indoor workouts to another level.

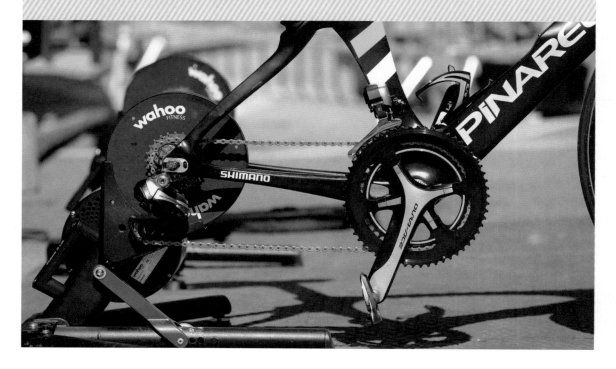

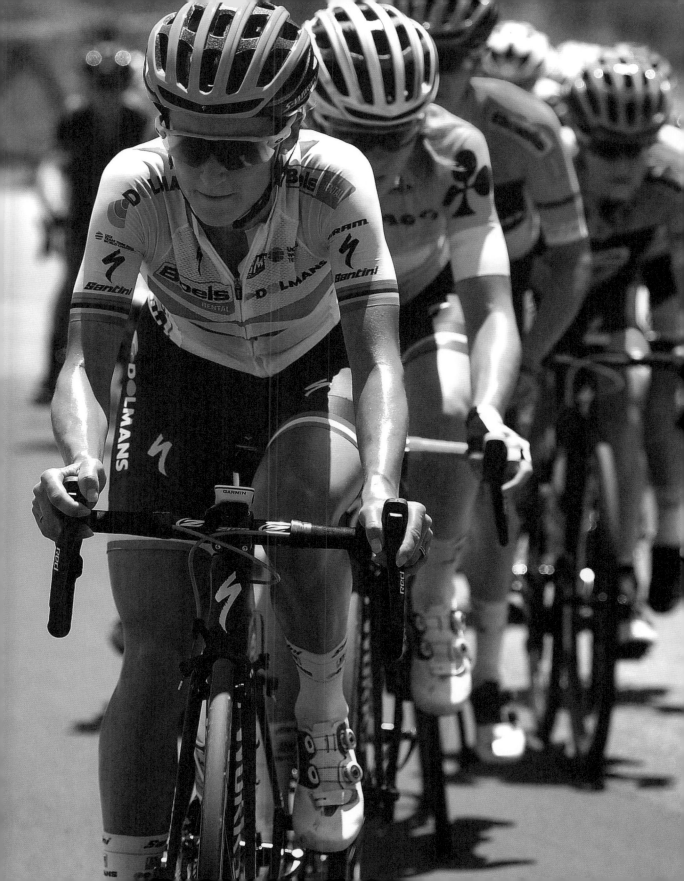

Special sessions

RECOVERY RIDES

Although much of it is anecdotal, there's fairly strong evidence that going out and riding the day after a tough training session or event can facilitate recovery. It helps to reduce the sensations of 'stiffening up' and DOMS (delayed onset muscle soreness). On the rest days of Grand Tours, the riders will normally head out for a couple of hours for this reason.

For a recovery ride to work, though, and not just add to your fatigue, it has to be done at genuine recovery pace/intensity. This has to be strict Zone 1, flat, small chainring, and no sensation of effort. You should imagine that your cranks are made of crystal and if you put any torque through them, they'll shatter. Fail to do this and you won't be achieving the intention of the ride.

If you think you'll struggle with the discipline required not to push and to let other riders overtake you, or you don't have suitable flat roads in your area, an indoor trainer or rollers can provide a recovery ride option. If you can't control yourself indoors, maybe recovery rides aren't for you and the sofa would be a better option.

Session duration: 30–60 mins

What is it? Easy recovery ride.
Why? To facilitate recovery the day after a hard training session or event.
When? Any time of year.
Notes: Has to be strict Zone 1 with no sensation of effort.
Warm-up: n/a

Main set
30–60 mins Zone 1, small chainring on flat roads

Cool-down: n/a

PRE-EVENT RIDE

Although it may seem counter-intuitive to head out for a ride the day before an event, it can help prevent your legs feeling stale and heavy. Spinning your legs out is an especially good idea if you've had a taper week or two and then travelled, and it's also a chance to give your bike a final check over. Like the recovery ride, it's predominately strict Zone 1, but to give your legs a bit of a reminder of what you'll be expecting from them the next day, some low resistance spin-up efforts are also included. This session is also suitable as a midweek workout during recovery weeks or in the final week before a key event.

Session duration: 40–60 mins

What is it? A ride for the day before an important event.
Why? To prevent legs feeling stale and heavy after tapering and travel.
When? Any time of year.
Notes: If you're unsure whether there will be suitable flat roads, rollers are ideal for this session.

Warm-up: 20 mins Zone 1 easy spinning

Main set
30 secs
- In low gear spin and staying seated, spin up to maximum cadence you can manage without bouncing
- Back off slightly and hold for rest of 30 seconds

2 mins Zone 1 easy spinning
Repeat for a total of 4–8 repetitions (after your final 30-second effort, go straight into cool-down)

Cool-down: Rest of session Zone 1 easy spinning

CARBOHYDRATE-FASTED RIDE

Carbohydrate-fasted rides have received a fair amount of attention, being credited as a key component of Sir Bradley Wiggins's training regime and weight loss before the 2012 Tour de France. They're not actually a new idea, though, with riders such as Sean Yates heading out on epic endurance rides fuelled only by a tablespoon of olive oil.

The theory behind carbohydrate-fasted training is that, by depriving the body of its preferred fuel, you force it to utilise your fat reserves. By doing so, your body becomes more efficient at using fat as a fuel and, in turn, you become a more efficient rider. By being able to use fat more effectively, you spare your carbohydrate stores and are less reliant on the carbohydrates you take in. This means that, during long events, you operate on less of a nutritional knife edge and, in simple terms, are able to ride faster for longer. We'll delve more into the physiological reasons behind this in Chapter 6.

One important thing to realise is that carbohydrate-fasted rides, despite what has been written about Sir Bradley, are not about weight loss or especially useful for it. Because you're effectively removing the body's energy source for higher intensity activity, namely carbohydrates, you're limited to Zones 1 and 2, so the actual calorie burn for the session will be relatively low. It's important, though, not to try to push harder than this as, along with negating the fat utilisation and fat burning adaptation benefits of the session, you'll find yourself coming to a grinding halt very quickly.

The best time for carbohydrate-fasted training is first thing in the morning, when your blood glucose is at its lowest. You can have black coffee or black tea before heading out, as caffeine can help with fat mobilisation. You can also take on some protein, such as scrambled eggs or some yoghurt, which, as you'll only be riding in Zones 1 and 2, you should be able to tolerate. This helps to prevent that empty stomach sensation and there's some evidence to suggest that taking on protein before and during such sessions can aid recovery. Stick strictly to Zones 1 and 2 and aim to ride for 30–120 minutes, depending on fitness and adaptation levels. Build up gradually if you're new to this type of training, as different riders' response and ability to cope with it varies. It can be a good idea to put a gel in your pocket just in case you misjudge it. You can also have a protein drink with you and sip on this during your ride. You should aim to have your full breakfast as soon as you get back from the ride.

A morning commute is a great opportunity to incorporate some carbohydrate-fasted rides into your training but remember the strict limit of Zones 1 and 2, and don't allow yourself to get sucked into any 'commuter racing'. Another option you can try in the early off season is to make the first 90–120 minutes of your weekend endurance ride carbohydrate-fasted. If you time this to end at a café, you can give your blood sugar a boost with a flapjack, for example, and then you'll finish the ride fuelling normally.

Session duration: 30–120 mins

What is it? Carbohydrate-fasted training.
Why? To develop your body's ability to utilise fat reserves as a fuel.
When? Off season.
Notes: As training load will be low, it can be used as the morning component of a two-session split day, with a higher intensity workout in the evening.

Warm-up: 10 mins Zone 1 easy spinning

Main set
10–100 mins
• Strict Zones 1 and 2
• Aim to predominately hold low–mid Zone 2

Cool-down: 10 mins Zone 1 easy spinning

How to improve your cycling performance

Have a goal/purpose for every ride

Whether it's recovery or a gruelling interval set, make sure that every ride has a clear and definite purpose and that you're not just accumulating junk miles for the sake of it. Have the plan and goals for the ride in your mind and try to stick to them. If you're just heading out for a 'ride' with your friends, be honest that it's probably not training but still needs to be factored into your training load and might impact on your priority sessions.

Don't avoid the sessions you dislike

If you find a session you particularly dislike, chances are it's addressing an area of your cycling fitness that needs work. We all prefer to do things that we're good at but it's often by working on our weaknesses that we stand to make the biggest gains. Remember that if a particular session fills you with absolute dread, there's normally a way to rejig the efforts to make it slightly more palatable without impacting too much on its effectiveness. You're always better off doing a modified workout than not doing any session at all!

Warm up and cool down

A structured warm-up is essential to prepare you physiologically and psychologically for a workout or a race. Warming up is proven to improve your performance, meaning you'll do better in races and get more out of your training. There's no need to go overboard – 20 minutes is plenty – but don't neglect it. Similarly, a cool-down allows your body and mind to return gradually to its pre-riding state. Use it to reflect on what you've just done and, as well as being the end of your current session, it's also the start of your next.

Midweek workouts

Prioritise two of these workouts each week, allowing an easier day before and after each of them. These sessions are sacrosanct and nothing, either non-cycling factors or additional rides, should impact on their quality. As a general rule, choose longer duration and lower intensity intervals in the off season and move on to the higher intensity efforts as you move into pre-season and season.

Long rides

Your long rides should be governed by your goals. If you're training for long sportives, then you will need to be getting in those 4-hour-plus rides. However, if your focus is shorter events, such as circuit racing, track or cyclo-cross, 2–3 hours is probably plenty. Pure base endurance rides have a place, early in the off season or during an easier recovery week, but if you have limited training time, you'll get more from these rides by including some focused higher intensity effort within them. These efforts should mirror your midweek workouts.

Recovery rides

For recovery rides to be worthwhile and effective, they have to be at genuine recovery pace. If you push harder than Zone 1, it's not a recovery ride. You won't be facilitating recovery and, in fact, you'll just be adding fatigue with the worst type of junk miles.

▶ Always question why you're doing a ride and what you're aiming to get out of it. Don't waste precious pedalling time.

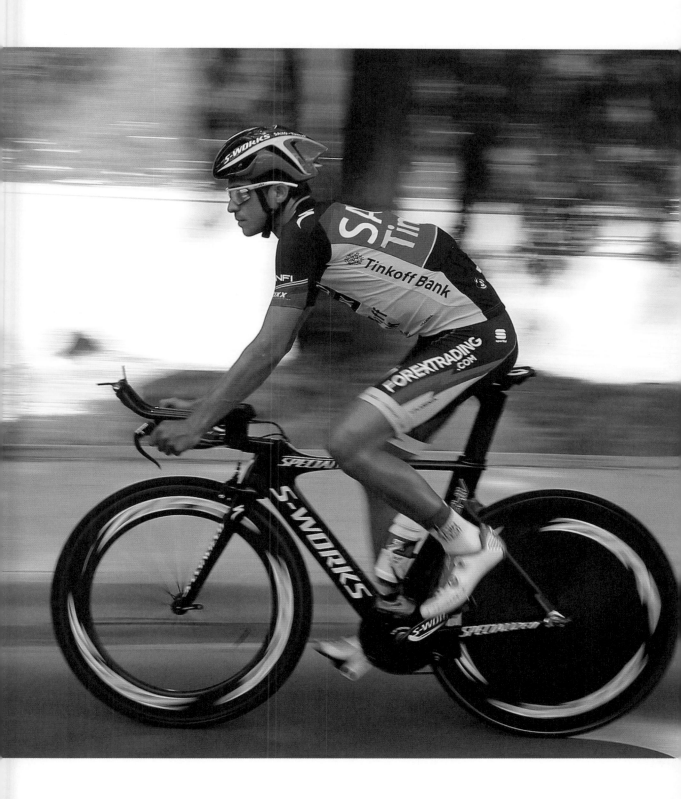

5 OFF THE BIKE TRAINING

OFF THE BIKE TRAINING WILL HELP TO MAKE YOU A MORE ROUNDED AND INJURY-RESILIENT CYCLIST, AS WELL AS BOOSTING YOUR PERFORMANCE AND MAKING YOU MORE COMFORTABLE ON THE BIKE.

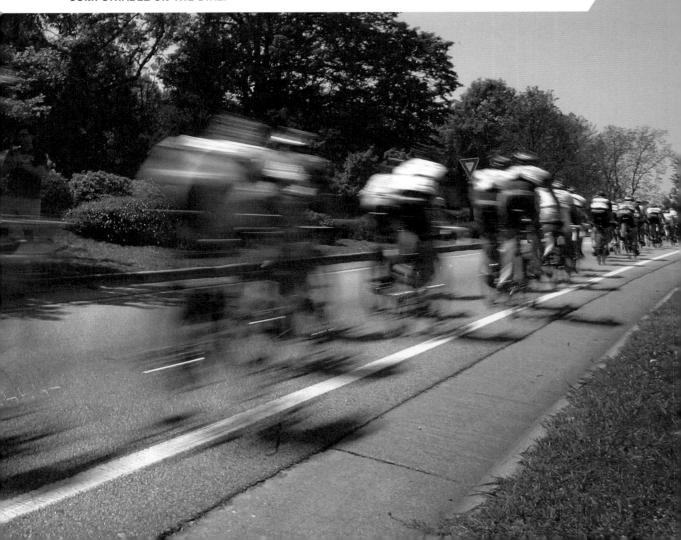

'Training can be monotonous, and it is hard work, but you never lose sight of why you're doing it. Every single effort of every single session counts in the months and years leading up to a big event.' **SIR CHRIS HOY**, ELEVEN-TIME WORLD CHAMPION AND SIX-TIME OLYMPIC CHAMPION

ONE OF THE FUNDAMENTAL PRINCIPLES of training is specificity. This simply states that the best training for a given activity is performing that activity. So, the best training for cycling is, unsurprisingly, getting out and turning those pedals over. It may seem contradictory, therefore, especially if the time that you can devote to training is limited, to suggest that you devote some of it to off the bike training.

The 'only worthwhile training for cycling is cycling' mindset prevailed within the sport until very recently and even now, within less progressive professional teams, the benefit of off the bike training is viewed with scepticism. Not so long ago the only 'cross training' that riders would do might be some cross-country skiing at the off-season get-together training camp. The shift in mindset embracing off the bike training was due in no small part to the work of the Great Britain Cycling Team in the build-ups to the Beijing and London Olympics.

Strength training had been an accepted component of track sprinters' training for years. In fact, they're often jokingly referred to as weightlifters who occasionally ride bikes. With certain track endurance disciplines, specifically the Team Pursuit, evolving to demand more sprint-type performance, the coaches started to prescribe more gym work for the endurance riders. The results were good and the riders started to notice improvements in others areas of their riding too, including on the road. The riders and coaches took this knowledge to their pro road teams, and slowly it became an accepted part of the training routine for most road cyclists.

▼ One of the biggest changes in the way pro cyclists train has been the inclusion of focused off the bike training.

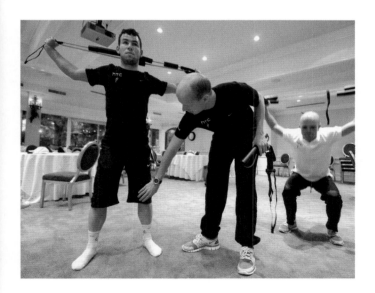

'I'd always do some gym work as I came off my post season break in October or November through to when I started racing in February. It'd always hurt like hell for the first few weeks but it definitely helped and made me stronger on the bike. I'd work with a personal trainer to ensure I was doing it right and, as the season drew nearer, I'd focus more on explosive plyometric type work to improve my sprint.'
DEAN DOWNING, EX-PRO, FORMER BRITISH CIRCUIT RACE CHAMPION AND NOW COACH

'Over the years I've focused a lot more on off the bike training. I've noticed that it has benefitted my stability, strength and explosive power on the bike. I'll do other activities sometimes, such as occasionally go for a run or do some paddle boarding, that's my idea of cross training, but the gym work is the important stuff.

TIFFANY CROMWELL, CANYON/SRAM

Off the bike training, if done correctly, can be directly beneficial to your cycling. It can improve your peak power production and make you more stable and efficient when pedalling. It can help you to hold a more aerodynamic position and generally be more comfortable on the bike.

Almost more important, though, are the indirect benefits. Cycling, although a brilliant form of exercise, works your body in very limited and fixed patterns. This means that, although you can be incredibly strong on the bike, if you're challenged outside of these confines you expose yourself to injury risk. Whether it's gardening, lifting the shopping or your children out of the car or some DIY, a loading pattern that you're not used to can easily cause injury and result in time off the bike. Additionally, the biomechanical issues that arise from the amount of time we spend seated in modern life, whether working at a desk or driving, for example, are compounded by the hunched-over flexed position that cycling involves. The resulting tight hip flexors, stiff lower back and poorly functioning glutes can manifest in a number of problems both on and off the bike.

Former Great Britain Cycling Team lead physiotherapist Phil Burt talks about overall physical condition being analogous to a pyramid. Your specific cycling fitness forms the top tiers and capstone of the pyramid. The lower tiers and the base are represented by your all-round and general conditioning level. You should aim to make this base as broad as possible as your cycling fitness will then be built on solid foundations. If your base is narrow or non-existent, no matter how good your cycling fitness, it's unstable and likely to break down. One of the best ways to build that broad base is to include a variety of off the bike training in your programme.

Strength work

Many cycling training manuals would at this stage recommend a gym-based cycling-specific strength routine. It would probably include squats, leg presses and an assortment of upper body and 'core' exercises. However, having worked with experts such as Phil Burt and Martin Evans, former head of conditioning with the Great Britain Cycling Team, I feel that this one-size-fits-all approach is at best ineffective and, at worst, possibly dangerous. With restricted movement patterns resulting from everyday life and time on the bike, complex movements such as squats and deadlifts are inappropriate for the majority of endurance-focused cyclists. Lacking sufficient

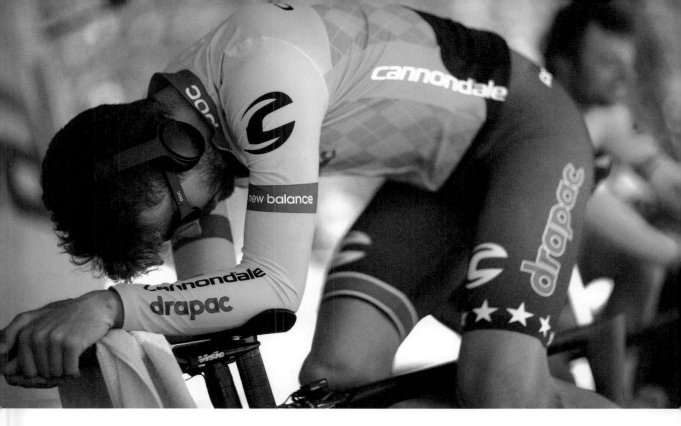

▲ Off the bike training can improve your cycling and make you more resistant to injury.

strength, range of movement and control, correct form is practically impossible. If you start adding load to poor form, it is almost guaranteed to lead to problems.

The construction and implementation of a cycling-specific strength routine should be highly individualistic and, as such, is beyond the remit of this book. I would strongly recommend *Strength and Conditioning for Cyclists* by Phil Burt and Martin Evans. Through an assessment based on the one used by the Great Britain Cycling Team, your weaknesses are identified and the optimum exercises to correct them recommended. It's a process that I've been through and highly recommend following. Even Olympic gold medal winners have to go through it on a regular basis. One of the basic tests is an active straight leg raise, which assesses hamstring, hip and lower back mobility. Sprinter Callum Skinner has to undertake and pass this test before every lifting session in the gym. If he fails the test, he has a series of mobilisation exercises, similar to those described below, to perform to get him through it and ready to lift. The support team know that if he attempts to lift without doing this, it significantly increases his injury risk and reduces the effectiveness of the workout. If, on any given day, the mobility exercises fail to give him a pass, maybe

'Off the bike training is really important as it's an unnatural and extremely demanding task for the body to sit on the bike for hours. During the training camp in December we analyse and assess all the riders to determine their weaknesses and what needs working on. We'll then give them exercises to do and a plan to follow.'

JULIA SCHULZE, TEAM DOCTOR, CANYON/SRAM

due to having worked particularly hard the day before, his training will be modified to accommodate this.

At the very least, if you're wanting to embark on a strength block, you should consult with a qualified fitness or health professional. You should explain your cycling goals to them and they should be able to help you to construct a suitable routine and demonstrate good technique.

Scheduling in strength work

If you already have a strength routine that you're happy with and are confident in your form and technique or are working with a qualified fitness professional, the best time to work on building strength is during the early off season. You won't be looking to perform very high-intensity sessions on the bike and therefore the additional fatigue from lifting can be accommodated. I would recommend scheduling in your strength sessions on the days following your midweek workouts or, if you're able to do a split day, do the bike session in the morning and the gym in the evening. This will allow for maximum recovery after the strength work so that the impact on the quality of your

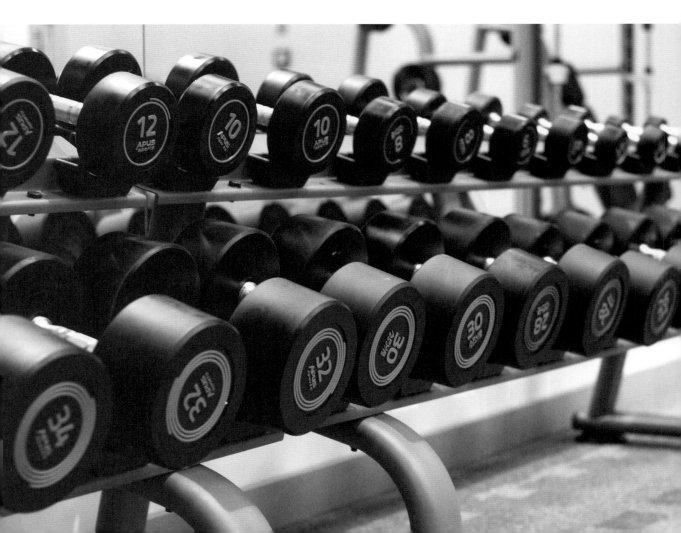

riding is minimal. Examples of how to schedule strength work into your training are given below. As you can see, to fit in three strength sessions a week, split days are your only real option.

To make gains, you should be looking to lift 2–3 times each week during your first early off season 8–12-week training block. As you move into late off season and pre-season, you should drop the number of strength sessions to 1–2 each week, with more of a focus on maintenance rather than progress. Be sure to monitor the impact it's having on your cycling workouts and, if necessary, back off the strength work more. During the season or in the run-up to an important event, you should probably be looking to drop to a single maintenance session each week or to remove the strength work completely from your routine.

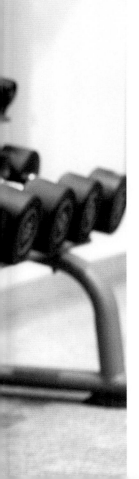

▼ The off-season is usually the best time to schedule in some focused strength training.

OFF SEASON X2 STRENGTH SESSIONS PER WEEK

Monday	**Big Gear/Low Cadence**
Tuesday	Strength
Wednesday	Rest
Thursday	Big gear/low cadence
Friday	Strength
Saturday	Endurance ride
Sunday	Rest

OFF SEASON X3 STRENGTH SESSIONS PER WEEK USING SPLIT DAYS

	AM	**PM**
Monday	Rest	Rest
Tuesday	Big gear/low cadence	Strength
Wednesday	Rest	Rest
Thursday	Big gear/low cadence	Strength
Friday	Rest	Rest
Saturday	Strength	Rest
Sunday	Endurance ride	

The myth of low weight/high rep for endurance

One of the most common mistakes that cyclists make when strength training is to think that, as they're endurance athletes, they should be lifting low weights for a high number of reps. They believe that sets of 20–50 reps best mimic the demands of cycling and so will result in the most transferable gains. Unfortunately, this is incorrect as even riding for as little as 30 minutes at an average cadence of 90 rpm will involve 2,700 pedal rotations. Even 3–5 sets of high rep lifting will come nowhere close to this number, so the idea of it mimicking the activity just doesn't tally. Also, for developing strength, high reps and low weight are practically useless. Lower rep ranges, typically 6–10 reps using appropriate load, are far more effective and beneficial.

Some riders also avoid lifting heavier weights because they're concerned about developing unnecessary bulk. This isn't a problem, as even bodybuilders who are lifting and eating with the sole intention of gaining bulk often struggle, unless unusually genetically blessed, to gain significant mass. Additionally, as you'll be combining strength work with cycling, known as concurrent training, this severely limits the potential for significant muscle growth.

Mobility work

One of the main requirements for having that broad base of conditioning is good mobility and flexibility beyond that required by cycling alone. Many riders are aware of stretching and maybe do some token stretches after a ride but it's normally fairly unfocused and without structure. Similarly, a lot of cyclists will occasionally dig out a foam roller but often only when feeling stiff or sore.

Mobility work combines tool-assisted self manual therapy (TASMT), using a foam roller or trigger ball to release an area, with stretching to work it through an extended range of motion. Almost all cyclists would benefit from focused mobility work throughout the year. It will help to address imbalances and tightness both from cycling and from daily life. It can improve your comfort and position on the bike and increase your resilience to injury from movements and activities outside of cycling.

Unlike strength training, mobility work will not have an acute negative impact on subsequent cycling workouts. In fact, you will probably find it makes you feel better on the bike. This means that you can schedule in mobility work at any time, even daily and on 'rest days', throughout the entire cycling year.

The routine suggested below takes just over 30 minutes to complete and covers most of the classic areas where both cycling and 'desk time' can cause problems. The more you can do of this type of work the better, really, but you should aim at the minimum for 2–3 focused bouts each week. You will probably find certain pairs of exercises feel tougher and that may indicate an area that needs working on. There's no reason why you can't work on certain movements daily or even multiple times per day.

CIRCUIT CLASSES AND CROSS-FIT

Circuit classes, boot camp and Cross-Fit can offer a motivating and convenient option for riders looking to incorporate some off the bike training into their routine, but although there's no doubt that group classes can be good for pushing yourself, they should be approached with caution. Often form and proper technique are neglected in favour of forcing out a few more reps and, with a high number of participants for the instructor to supervise, little coaching or correction can be given. It's unlikely that the class will be cycling specific and although there might be some injury/exercise history screening beforehand, the class won't be tailored or significantly modified to your needs. Finally, classes of this nature tend to err on the side of low weight and high reps and, as previously discussed, the benefit of this is questionable.

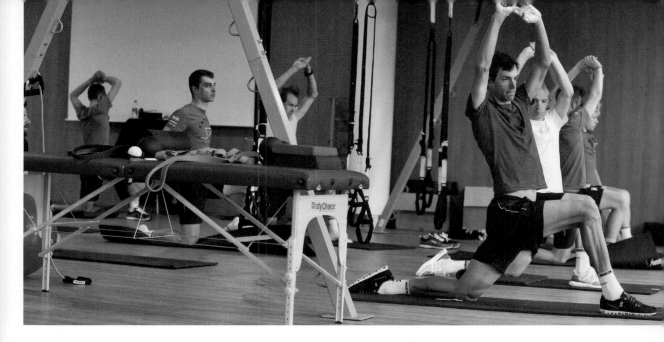

▲ Restorative off the bike work, such as mobility training, yoga and Pilates, should be a staple throughout the year.

The advice always given previously for traditional stretching routines was immediately post-exercise. However, the last thing you want to do when you come in cold and wet from a long hard ride or dripping with sweat from a gruelling session on the turbo is roll around on a mat. It's uncomfortable and you're unlikely to do a decent job. You're better off getting clean, warm and fed, and then dedicating some quality time to mobility work. In fact, you can work on this routine at any time, even in front of the television in the evening. My preference tends to be first thing in the morning a few times a week for the full routine and then 'as and when' working on particular exercises when I feel I need them.

You'll need to purchase a foam roller. The hollow ones are really good as they're light for travelling and you can pack gear inside them. You'll also need a trigger point ball. You don't need anything special – a hockey ball or a firm rubber dog ball are both perfect.

The A) exercise is always TASMT.
- Whether using the foam roller or trigger point ball, don't just roll backwards and forwards. Explore the area you're working on, shift your body weight around to change the emphasis and, when you find tight spots, oscillate over them until they release.
- Spend at least 2 minutes on each area or side before moving on.

The B) exercise is always a stretching movement.
- Move and develop the stretch, don't just hold it passively.
- Once you find the limit of your movement or a tight area, breathe deeply and try to work through it.
- Hold and develop each stretch for 2 minutes.

1A) QUAD FOAM ROLL

This muscle group at the front of your thighs consists of four muscles: the rectus femoris, vastus lateralis, vastus medialis and sartorius. The rectus femoris especially is responsible for driving your pedals around but, if allowed to become too tight, can have an adverse effect on both posture and biomechanics, resulting in lower back pain and, potentially, hip and knee problems.

- Lie face down in a front plank position with one thigh on the roller.
- Bend the knee of the leg being rolled and hook it behind the ankle of the other leg to hold it in position.
- Roll up and down the full length of your thigh from the top of your hips to just above your knee.
- Rotate your body from side to side to focus more on the inner and outer thigh.
- Repeat with the other leg.

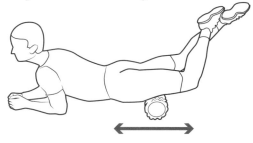

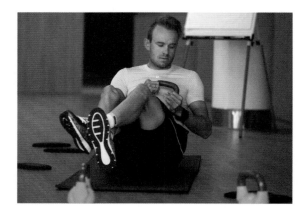

1B) KNEELING HIP FLEXOR STRETCH

- From a kneeling position, bring your right leg forward so that you're in a kneeling lunge. You may find it more comfortable if your left knee is on a towel or mat.
- Make sure your right knee is directly over the right ankle and that your upper body is tall with your centre of gravity over your kneeling left knee.
- Contract your trunk muscles without arching your back, squeeze your glutes and lean forward, increasing the flexion of your right leg and creating a stretch on your left hip and thigh.
- Allow the stretch to develop and intensify it by moving further forwards or by trying it with the rear leg elevated.
- Repeat with the other leg.

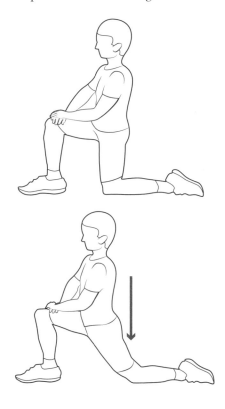

◄ Consistency is the key with mobility work. 5 minutes every day is better than an hour every now and then.

2A) GLUTE TRIGGER POINT BALL

When functioning properly, the muscles in your backside should play a significant role in an even and powerful pedal stroke. However, for many cyclists, poorly firing glutes due to tightness means less power and more load placed on your already overworked quads.

- In a seated position, with your hands providing support behind, place the ball under one of your buttocks.
- Cross the leg of that side so that its ankle is on the knee of the other leg.
- Tilt your body weight slightly towards the side you're working on.
- Work over the entire buttock, rolling the ball about and shifting your body weight.
- Repeat on the other side.

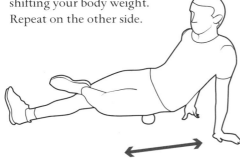

'Functional strength training for the legs is also important to help prevent injuries and to build muscle mass. It's more of an off-season focus though as, because it's very demanding and exhausting, it's hard to schedule into the in season without having a detrimental effect on race performance. For this reason, general mobility work and trunk strengthening is better throughout the year.'

ANDREAS LANG, TEAM PHYSIOLOGIST, CANYON/SRAM

2B) PIGEON POSE

- Kneel on all fours and then bring your right leg through, placing it flat on the floor between your hands, with a 90-degree bend at the knee.
- Extend your left leg out behind you, rotating your knee so that your knee and toes are on the floor.
- Sit back into the stretch, aiming for a straight and level pelvis. Your navel should be in line with the inside of your left thigh.
- Lift your chest up and breathe through the stretch.
- Experiment with dropping your chest down towards the floor and, adding more rotation, gently work back and forth through any restrictions.
- Change sides.

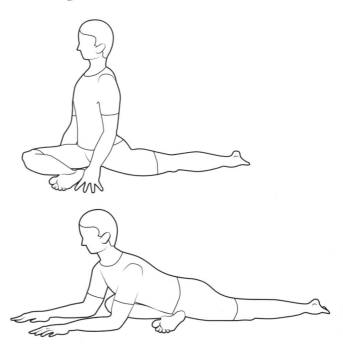

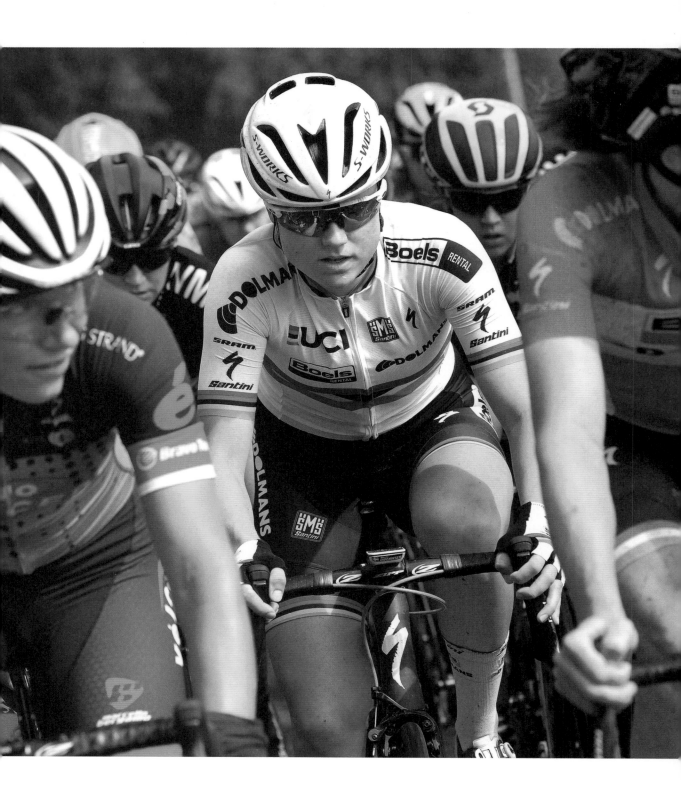

3A) HAMSTRING FOAM ROLLER

Sitting on a bike or at a desk or driving can cause the hamstrings to tighten. This can make holding an aero position on the bike difficult and is one of the most common causes of lower back pain on the bike.

- In a seated position, with your hands behind you for support, position either a foam roller or a trigger point ball under the mid-point of the back of your thigh.
- Cross one ankle over the other to focus all your weight on one leg.
- Roll up and down, rotating your body to hit the inner and outer thigh and reposition the ball or roller as necessary.
- Change sides and work on the other hamstring.

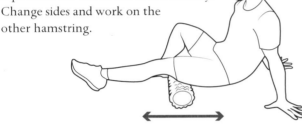

3B) LYING HAMSTRING STRETCH

- Lie on your back and loop a strap or towel around your left foot.
- Bring your knee towards your chest.
- Apply tension to your hamstring by straightening your knee. Increase the intensity by bending and straightening your leg.
- Repeat with the other leg.

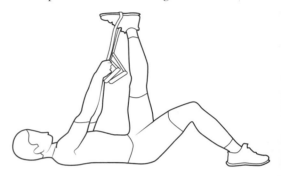

4A) PEC TRIGGER BALL

With the hunched-over posture associated with cycling and keyboard work, tightness through the chest can easily develop. This can result in rounded shoulders and knock-on problems with your neck. By relaxing your chest muscles, you'll bring your shoulders back and relax your thoracic region.

- Lying on your front, position the trigger point ball so that it's nestled below your collar bone in the soft tissue between your shoulder and breast bone.
- Bend the arm on that side to 90 degrees. Have your other arm straight by your side or bent with your hand under your forehead.
- Rotate your head to look in the other direction and rest it on the mat.
- Gently extend the bent arm and return it to the bent position, pausing and working on any tight areas.
- Repeat on the other side.

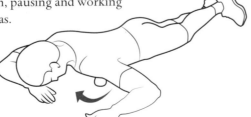

4B) PEC STRETCH

- Stand in a doorway and, with your arm bent to 90 degrees, place your forearm against the frame.
- Develop a stretch across your chest by leaning into the frame and rotating away from it.
- Repeat on the other side.

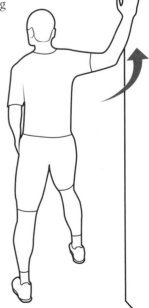

Yoga and Pilates

Both yoga and Pilates can be excellent complementary activities to cycling, developing both mobility and functional strength. Performed well under good instruction, they can both definitely contribute to that broad conditioning base and are ideal activities throughout the cycling year.

There are many forms of yoga: Bikram in a heated studio, the very gentle hatha and the extremely demanding ashtanga, to name a few. You may even be able to find a class specifically aimed at cyclists. As with all classes, quality of instruction is key and, with yoga, even the smallest adjustments can make a huge difference to the quality, intensity and effectiveness of a pose. It's worth looking for some smaller classes at a dedicated yoga centre or even investing in some initial one-to-one instruction. Talk to the instructor about your cycling and they should be able to recommend specific poses or sequences that will be beneficial to you. You may have to try a number of classes and styles before you find one that suits, but it's definitely worth persevering. Like the mobility routine, yoga is an off the bike activity that you can work on throughout the year without having to worry about any acute detrimental effects on the quality of your training on the bike. It's also good for developing breathing control and some riders swear that this transfers over to their riding.

Pilates is named after its founder, Joseph Pilates, who originally developed it while in an internment camp during the First World War as a holistic exercise system for mind and body. Since then it became popular firstly with dancers, who used it for rehabilitation from injury, and then with the wider exercising public. Like yoga, if you find the right class and instructor, it can be brilliant for developing both mobility and strength and is an excellent complementary activity to cycling. You should try to find a dedicated Pilates centre and, if possible, find a small class using reformers. These are the wooden-framed devices that utilise springs to provide resistance to the movements you perform. Working on one of these with a knowledgeable instructor is a million miles from a mat-based 'Pilates class' at your local leisure centre.

Running

For many cyclists, running is a dirty word, but it can be a useful cross-training option. If you only have a spare half hour at lunchtime, the weather makes cycling unsafe or you are travelling without your bike, popping on a pair of running shoes can be a time-effective way of keeping your fitness topped up. Minute for minute, it also tends to burn more calories than cycling so if weight loss is a priority for you, it can be a good choice. However, especially if you're not used to it, it can be extremely fatiguing for your legs and has to be carefully scheduled so as not to impact negatively on your cycling sessions. As with strength training, the best time of year for running is during the off season when your cycling sessions aren't so demanding. Schedule any running into your training week to allow maximum recovery between it and your next cycling session.

▶ Yoga and Pilates can both be excellent complementary activities to cycling.

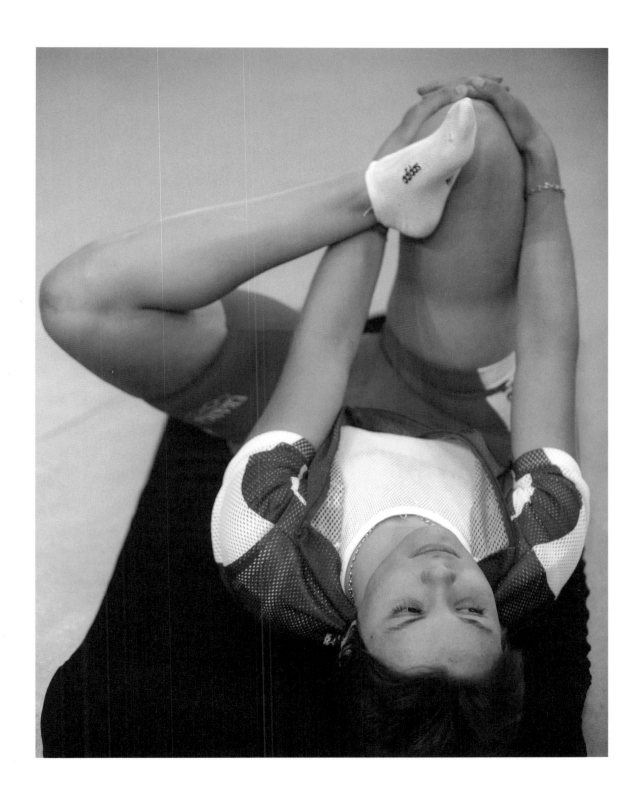

You should try if possible to run off-road rather than pounding tarmac. It's not so much the impact that you're trying to avoid but the extremely repetitive foot strikes that road running entails. Off-road, every foot strike will be different and, because you're having to focus on avoiding roots, rocks and the like, your running form will tend to be better too. Fartlek, Swedish for 'speed play', is a form of unstructured interval training that can work well and provide variety of intensity when running on the trails. In its purest form, you run hard when you feel strong, back off to recover and then go again. You can, however, use landmarks (such as a certain tree) to sprint to, or say you're going to attack every hill, or even work on a minute on/minute off principle. What you're looking for, though, is to mix up the pace and avoid mindless plodding. Be sure to spend at least 10 minutes warming up with steady jogging and then the same at the end of the session as a cool-down, with a couple of minutes of walking to finish.

It's no coincidence that a number of top cyclo-cross racers in the UK, including Nick Craig and Rob Jebb, are also highly accomplished fell runners. Cyclo-cross obviously involves some running and the steep climbs and descents involved in fell running provide a brilliant crossover for the high intensity stop-go nature of cyclo-cross racing. Cyclo-cross legend Niels Albert includes at least one running workout in his training throughout most of the season. It's very sprint focused, mimicking the short run-ups typically found on a cross course, and, so as not to cause too much fatigue and muscle damage, never more than 30 minutes in length.

Swimming

Swimming can be the perfect 'recovery day' activity, involving zero impact on your legs and with the pressure of the water actually having therapeutic recovery benefits. Australian pro Richie Porte came from a swimming and triathlon background, and still includes significant swim work in his training schedule during the off season. He's especially convinced of the benefits on his breathing capacity. There's no reason, if you enjoy a swim, that it can't be part of your routine throughout the year. It shouldn't have any negative effects on your cycling training and therefore shouldn't present any scheduling issues.

Rowing

Another great cross-training activity for cyclists is rowing and it's no coincidence that a number of former rowers, Rebecca Romero for Great Britain and Cameron Wurf for Australia being two, have succeeded as cyclists both on the track and on the road. Also, Sir Bradley Wiggins is currently dabbling with going the other way, from cycling to rowing. Both activities are non-impact and, for cyclists, the recruitment of the upper body means it's excellent for developing better all-round conditioning. It's also very good for warming up the entire body prior to any strength work.

How to improve your cycling performance

Build a broad base

Although there are proven direct benefits of off the bike training for your cycling, the main reason for doing it is to develop a broad base of conditioning and make yourself more robust and less susceptible to injury. Both cycling and everyday life, especially time spent seated, can cause postural issues and imbalances, and countering these should be a priority. It's worth investing some time in off the bike training for this reason and to reduce the likelihood of enforced time off the bike due to injury.

Strength work

Strength work in the gym can be brilliant for cyclists but should be approached with caution. It has to be personalised and ideally supervised, at least initially, by a qualified professional. Focused strength work should be scheduled during the early off season when its impact on cycling workouts will be minimal. As you move into the pre-season and season, strength training should be reduced to a maintenance level or removed from the training plan entirely.

Mobility work

Combining tool-assisted self manual therapy (TASMT) and more traditional stretching techniques, mobility work is a must-do for all cyclists. Rather than being viewed as a post-cycling bolt-on, often given only token attention, a mobility routine should be a stand-alone part of your regular training. It can be done throughout the year and will have

▶ Don't just ride your bike. Include off the bike training to make you a more rounded and robust athlete

no negative effect on your cycling training. You'll probably find, in fact, that it improves your comfort, position and performance on the bike, and makes you feel less stiff and sore off it.

Other activities

Top of the list of beneficial cross training activities for the majority of cyclists are yoga and Pilates. If you don't have the discipline or self-motivation for mobility work at home, both of these are potentially ideal alternatives. Take the time to find the right class and instructor and even invest in some one-to-one tuition. Don't be scared of running, it can be a highly time-effective cross-training activity. However, get off-road and onto the trails, mix up your pace and be wary of the effect it can have on subsequent cycling sessions. Hitting the pool is great as a 'recovery activity' and might have benefits for your breathing capacity. Rowers seem to make great cyclists so, it can be a great option at the gym if you want a change from the bike.

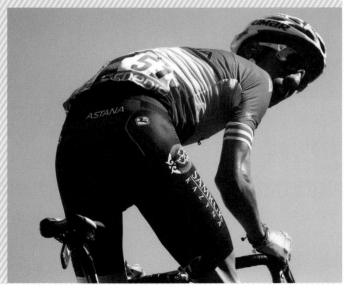

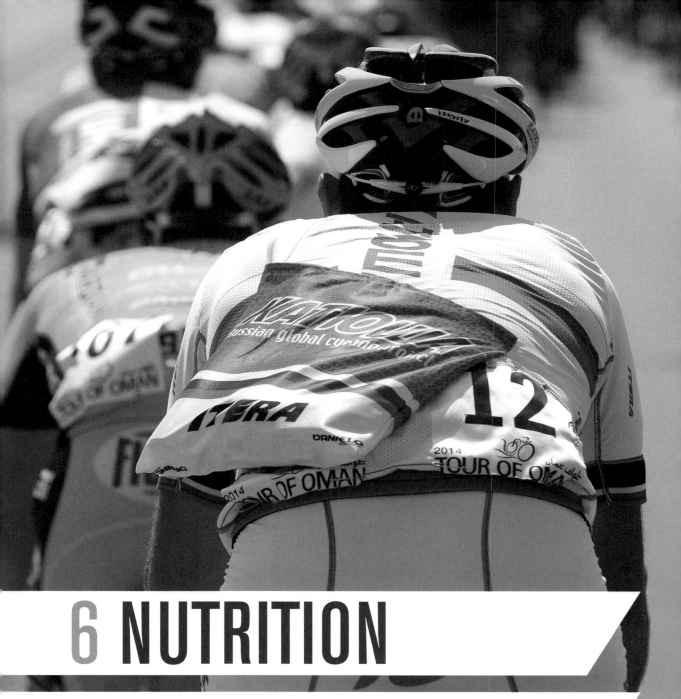

6 NUTRITION

IN THIS CHAPTER, WE OUTLINE THE FUNDAMENTALS OF FUELLING BOTH ON AND OFF THE BIKE. THIS IS A CRUCIAL AREA FOR MAXIMISING CYCLING PERFORMANCE, BUT ONE THAT MANY RIDERS GET WRONG.

'Too many riders focus solely on tangible sessions or second-shaving aerodynamic or lightweight kit. They miss out the fundamental of the fuel they provide for their engine. You wouldn't expect a car to run on the wrong type of fuel, so why would you expect your body to perform on the wrong type of fuel either?'

NIGEL MITCHELL, CANNONDALE-DRAPAC NUTRITIONIST AND FORMERLY WITH THE GREAT BRITAIN CYCLING TEAM AND TEAM SKY

GO ON ANY CYCLING FORUM and probably the most common subject for questions and debate is nutrition for cycling, both on and off the bike. Out of all the areas of cycling performance, this is probably the one most plagued by misunderstanding, misinformation, poor interpretation of science and dated concepts and beliefs. It's not so long ago, even at the highest level of the sport, that riders would be tucking into steak on the morning of a ride, avoiding drinking while on the bike and gorging themselves on huge plates of pasta. Fortunately, the science of sports nutrition has evolved hugely in recent years and now a dedicated nutritionist is a key member of any national or professional team. The importance of protein, the maintenance of gut health and personalised nutritional plans are all now seen by top riders as normal essentials rather than quirky fads.

Nutrition for performance cycling is a hugely detailed area and although we'll cover the essentials here, I'd strongly recommend further reading. Nigel Mitchell's book, *Fuelling the Cycling Revolution: The Nutritional Strategies Behind Grand Tour Wins and Olympic Gold Medals*, is the go-to resource.

As with all aspects of performance, nutrition is hugely individual. What might work brilliantly for one rider can be disastrous for another. It's essential that, along with following the recommendations in this and other books, you experiment in training and find what works best for you. Once you've found a strategy and products that suit you, stick with them and don't be tempted, especially on the day of a major event, to try something different.

The basics for a long ride

Whether it's a sportive, training ride or a long road race or time trial, the basics of pre-, during and post-ride nutrition are the same. The specific foods mentioned are just suggestions and might not work for you. The key is to take the amounts of carbohydrates and other macronutrients required, and to find food options that provide these and suit you.

The day before

◀ Correct fuelling is one of the most important factors in cycling performance.

Aim to eat normally the day before a big ride and not risk anything that may upset your stomach. Having probably tapered off training in the lead-up to the event, your body's own carbohydrate stores in your muscles and liver in the form of glycogen will already be fully loaded. This means there's no need for huge plates of pasta as, once your glycogen stores are full, you can't load any more in. In fact, eating too much the night before can leave you feeling bloated and uncomfortable the following morning. Steer clear of spicy food, hard to digest red meat and excessive amounts of fibre. Opt for a moderate serving of rice or pasta, some lighter protein, such as chicken or fish, and some salad.

Pre-ride

Working back from your ride start time, you should be looking to allow ideally 3 hours to digest your breakfast. If you know, though, that the ride is going to start off fairly steadily, you can reduce this time to between 90 minutes and 2 hours. You should be looking to consume approximately 1g carbohydrate per kg of body weight for your pre-ride breakfast. A 70g (2½oz) serving of porridge will provide you with about 40g (1½oz) of carbohydrates, and by chopping a banana into it and adding some honey, you can boost that by another 20–40g (¾–1½oz). It can also be a good idea to add some protein, such as a 2–3-egg omelette or some yoghurt, as this will slow the digestion, absorption and release of energy from the carbohydrates.

Have your regular morning cup of tea or coffee and keep sipping water or sports drink throughout the morning. Coffee is a key pre-ride ritual for many riders and it certainly has some performance benefits. It has been shown not only to increase awareness and lower perceived exertion but also to facilitate the mobilisation of fat reserves for fuel. However, there is still some debate whether, to really benefit from its boost, you need to abstain from habitual use. One of the main benefits of strong coffee for many riders, though, is to ensure that they have a bowel movement before heading out for a ride. Between your breakfast and heading out, you may also want to snack on bananas, energy bars or rice cakes, but don't overdo it and leave yourself feeling bloated.

On the bike

Your mantra for feeding on the bike should be little, often and early. You should be taking on food right from the start of a long ride, not waiting until you feel hungry. You've got to remember that you're not eating for that moment but for 15–20km (9–12 miles) down the road.

The goal is to consume 0.5–1g of

'The night before a race is just pasta and protein and salad. I don't have a massive breakfast and I'll aim to have it 3 hours before the race. I then like to keep nibbling the whole way up to it. I usually find if I eat too much for breakfast I'm uncomfortable for the morning, so that's not good. It works better for me to have a normal sized breakfast and then just snack the whole way up to the race, almost starting my on the bike feeding before I get on the bike.'

HANNAH BARNES, CANYON/SRAM

carbohydrates per kg of body weight each hour. This should be broken down into a micro-feed every 20–30 minutes.

For an 80kg (176lb) rider aiming to eat at the upper end of this range, this might consist of:

500ml (18fl oz) of sports drink mixed at 6%	= 30g (1oz)
1 gel	= 30g (1oz)
½ energy bar	= 15g (½oz)
Total	**= 75g (2½oz)**

For steadier paced riding, many riders prefer to eat 'real' food such as fig rolls, filled rolls or flapjacks. Just do the nutritional sums for the amount of carbohydrates they supply and it's easy to work out how much you need. If the pace or intensity increases, or you need a quicker boost, that's when you might want to turn to a gel.

'My issue is, if I have really tasty snacks in the house, I don't just eat them on the bike, I'll eat them the rest of the day! So I'll tend to only buy things that I'd only eat on the bike. Bananas and sometimes malt loaf, but that seizes your jaw together in the winter. My general remit is to go down the cereal bar aisle and pick whatever doesn't look too tasty but contains the right amount of carbs.' **KATIE ARCHIBALD**, GREAT BRITAIN CYCLING TEAM

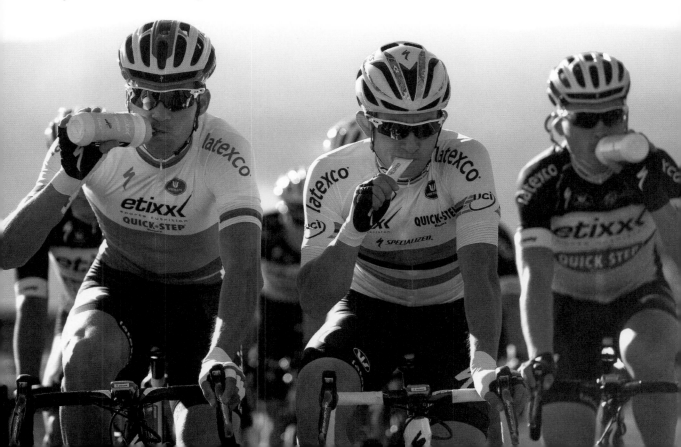

'During a race I aim for a bar or a gel every 45 minutes and a bottle. It varies a bit if it's hot or cold. If you wait until you feel hungry though and until you remember, it's often too late so I have to really remember to do it. Often during a race I'll try and eat as much as I can during the first couple of hours before the race hots up and hope that means I can get away with less regular feeds during the final hour or so. During those first two hours I'll normally eat solid food like bars, paninis or rice cakes. When it gets crazy I switch to gels for fast energy.' **HANNAH BARNES**, CANYON/SRAM

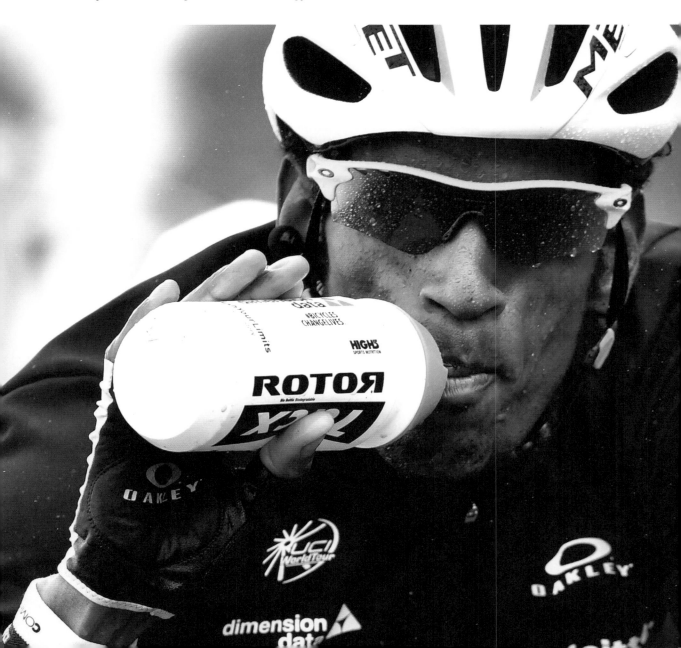

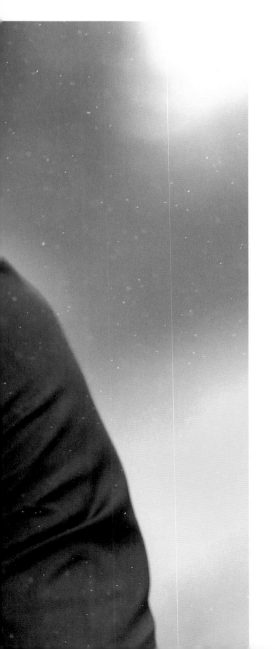

If you are having a café stop, remember to factor this in to your fuelling and try to opt for lighter and easily digestible options. A full cooked breakfast isn't a good idea if you know the ride pace will increase after the stop!

Be disciplined with your feeding right through to the end of the ride. Many riders make the mistake of skipping a final feed because they figure they only have a few kilometres left and it isn't worth it. It's not unusual, however, for the ride distance to be inaccurate, or there could be a climb you weren't expecting or you could take longer than expected due to a puncture or mechanical. Studies have shown that just by taking some carbohydrate solution into the mouth, performance increases and perceived exertion drops practically instantaneously. If you're suffering on a climb or struggling in the final few kilometres of a ride, it's always worth popping a gel or having a swig of sports drink for this boost.

Post-ride

Assuming that you've fuelled your ride well, you shouldn't be finishing it feeling ravenously hungry. Your priority is to get some protein into your system to kick-start your recovery, aiming to consume approximately 20g (¾oz). However, before you reach for that protein shake, ask yourself if you really need it. If you're not going to be able to eat for an hour or so, you've ridden for 90 minutes plus or especially hard, such as a 40km (25 mile) time trial, cyclo-cross race or intense interval session, a protein drink is a convenient option. However, don't make the mistake of doubling up by having a recovery drink and then sitting down to a full meal also. It's not going to help your recovery and it's certainly not going to do any favours for your waistline.

'After I cross the line, I always crave some soda and then, once I get back to the bus, I have a protein shake. The team have also normally made up some food. I've got a really really sweet tooth so they've normally made me sweet rice, which is rice, milk, cinnamon and honey, and I just mix it up with yoghurt and honey and fruit and nuts and stuff. Most people have just rice with mozzarella, pesto and tuna.' **HANNAH BARNES**, CANYON/SRAM

Pro race-day nutrition

Provided by Canyon/SRAM, this is an example of a typical racing day food diary for one of their riders. This would be for a 60kg (132lb) female rider.

4–5 hours before start: First breakfast (relatively low levels of fat and fibre)

- Fairly large serving (50–60g) of oat flakes or cereal made with water and with added dried fruit, nuts and seeds
- 2–3 slices of white bread with honey, jam and cream cheese
- 1–2 scrambled eggs
- Fruit, such as banana, kiwi, apple etc
- 1–2 cups of coffee or tea

2–3 hours before start: Second breakfast

- Serving of pasta or rice (50–100g/1¾–3½oz) with olive oil or light tomato sauce
- 0.3–0.5 litres (10–18fl oz) of mineral water or a mixture of mineral water and fruit juice

20–30 minutes before start

- 1 bottle of water (500ml) or isotonic drink
- 1 energy bar, rice cake or a panini with jam, cream cheese or banana

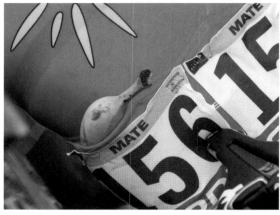

In jersey/on bike

- 2 bottles of isotonic drink (500ml each) or 1 bottle of isotonic drink and 1 bottle of water
- 2–3 energy bars
- 2–3 gels
- 2–3 paninis or rice cakes

▲ Try what other riders use but remember, we're all individuals so you've got to find what works for you.

During the race, the aim is to take on about 60–80g (2–2¾oz) of carbohydrates per hour along with 200ml (7fl oz) of liquid (6–10 per cent carbohydrates and 0.5–1g/l sodium) every 15 minutes. Whenever possible, try to eat 'real' food, saving gels for when the racing gets hard, and do not wait until you feel thirsty to have a drink. With each gel, try to drink at least 250ml of water.

Within 15–30 minutes of finish

- 500ml (18fl oz) recovery drink (60–80g/2–2¾oz carbohydrates, 20g/¾oz protein)

Within 90 minutes of finish

A Carbohydrate rich, protein moderate and low fat meal

- 500ml (18fl oz) of mineral water or a mixture of mineral water and fruit juice

Snack between race and dinner

- Cereal with fruit

Dinner

- Meat or fish (100g/3½oz), potatoes/rice/pasta/bread (100–200g/3½–7oz)

Pacing and fuelling

One of the crucial aspects when considering nutrition on the bike is the intrinsic link between your pace/riding intensity and your body's ability to digest and utilise fuel. We've already seen that, on a long ride, you should be aiming to consume 0.5–1g of carbohydrates per kg of body weight each hour. It's important to try not to exceed this amount as your body simply won't cope. It's also important to pace accurately as, if you try to go too hard and take on fuel, it just doesn't work.

Riders suffering digestive distress during long rides tend to blame the fuel they've taken on – 'It was a different gel to the ones I'm used to ...' – but in most cases it boils down to poor or overambitious pacing. If you're working too hard, your body will divert blood away from your digestive system and to your leg muscles. This effectively shuts down your digestive system, meaning any food already in your stomach will just sit there and you won't extract any nutrients or energy from it. As well as starting to feel bloated and nauseous, you're not providing your body with carbohydrates to fuel your riding and so you start to weaken. If you try to take on fuel to give yourself some energy, it just adds to the stockpile in your stomach, worsening the bloating and nausea.

Although, like most aspects of training and performance, there's considerable individual variance and some riders just seem to tolerate fuelling better, while others have ultra-sensitive stomachs, there are some decent guidelines to follow.

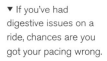

▼ If you've had digestive issues on a ride, chances are you got your pacing wrong.

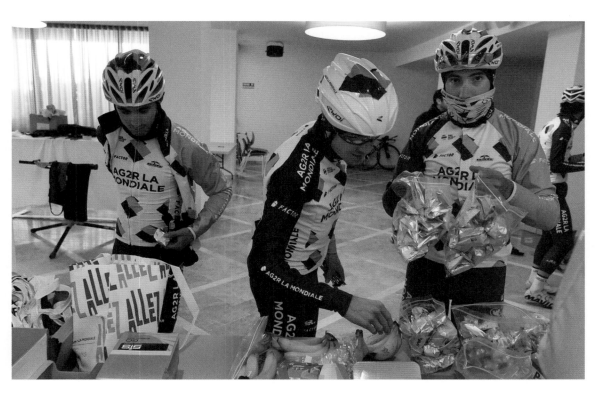

In general, for 'real' food such as bars, flapjacks, filled paninis, etc., you're looking at sticking within Zone 2 to be able to digest and process them. If you're pushing into Zone 3, you'll probably be more reliant on gels and sports drinks. Moving into Zone 4, and reaching your FTP/FTHR, you'll definitely be at that point where your digestive system will be going into shutdown.

This has a number of implications for training and pacing longer events. Try to use flat sections and downhills, when you'll be able to cruise along in Zones 1 and 2, to take on real food. Also, during the early stages of a training ride or event, the pace may be less intense and you should take advantage of this to fuel up.

On really long climbs, such as you might encounter in the Alps or Pyrenees, be really measured with your pacing, try to cap your effort to Zone 3 and switch to gels and energy drinks. For rides with multiple steeper climbs that force you over Zone 4, time your fuelling so you're not hitting them with loads of solid food sitting in your stomach. You'll often see pros with route crib notes taped to their stems. Do a bit of research about the route, note down the significant climbs, and adapt your fuelling strategy accordingly. You have to be flexible and, although you might want to take something on every 20 minutes, if that falls halfway up a 20 per cent cobbled climb, it's not the time to be reaching into your pocket for a snack!

Above all, the key thing is to practise your pacing and fuelling in training. That's the time to find out what you can tolerate and what you can't. It's then a case of applying what you've learned in training on event day and not getting sucked into trying to ride too hard for your ability.

FAT ADAPTATION AND CARBOHYDRATE-FASTED TRAINING

A lot of attention has been given to fat adaptation and carbohydrate-fasted training. As we've already discussed in Chapter 4, carbohydrate-fasted sessions, as long as they're conducted correctly, can be a good way to improve the body's ability to burn fat as a fuel and increase a rider's efficiency and endurance. For almost all riders, especially those targeting long events, increasing fat adaptation and reducing reliance on carbohydrates is a good idea. However, like many aspects of training and nutrition, fat adaptation has been misreported by both specialist cycling and non-cycling media, and misinterpreted by riders.

Chris Froome has been widely reported as advocating a low-carb diet and, although he probably does significantly reduce his carbohydrate intake at certain points in his training, when he ramps up the intensity, and certainly during any races, he definitely wouldn't be eating low carb.

No matter how well fat-adapted you are, once you push above a certain intensity, your body needs carbohydrates. Fail to provide them and you'll come to a grinding halt. If all your riding is going to be strict Zones 1 and 2 steady pace, you might be able to get away with a full-time low-carb approach but, if you're looking to up the pace, you're going to need some carbs.

Fuel the session

Developing the concept of what we've just discussed regarding fat adaptation, a simple and seemingly obvious but often overlooked nutritional rule is to fuel the session you're planning to do. For example, if you've got a long endurance ride with some higher intensity efforts planned, you're going to need a fairly carbohydrate-rich breakfast and a big bowl of porridge would be appropriate. However, if you're on a recovery day, you don't need all of those carbohydrates, and a smaller and more protein/fat-focused breakfast, such as an omelette, would be better. Similarly, for midweek workouts, assuming you'll be completing them in the evening, you don't need a huge carbohydrate-rich breakfast or a huge lunch. Sensible eating along with a snack, such as a banana or a flapjack/energy bar, an hour or so before and maybe, if it's a really tough session, a gel midway through or some sports drink, would suffice. We've already discussed when a dedicated recovery drink is necessary and you certainly don't need one after every ride.

In summary, if you're eating similar meals every day regardless of the riding you're doing, it's very likely that you're either under-fuelling or, more likely, chronically over-fuelling your training. When you plan your training, also plan your meals to complement it.

Understanding a bonk

You're taking part in a sportive and, despite pushing a little harder than you would on a training ride, 4 hours in you're feeling good and riding strong. You've been feeding well and, with just an hour of riding to go, you only have one more significant climb to tackle. You hit the bottom of the climb and, as expected and planned, your heart rate rises, hitting upper Zone 3 and even tickling the bottom of Zone 4. It's not a problem, though, as you've been riding hills all day at that intensity and you popped a gel at the foot of the climb. Halfway up, though, you suddenly start to weaken, and, in just a few more pedal strokes, your vision closes in, you feel a cold sweat and you can barely maintain forward progress. You've bonked, had a 'fringale' as the French would say, encountered the 'man with his hammer' or, scientifically, entered a state of exercise-induced hypoglycaemia or low blood sugar level.

The good news is you're certainly not alone and it's something that has happened to almost all cyclists, even the best in the world on the biggest stage. On Stage 18 of the 2013 Tour de France, Chris Froome suffered a potentially race-losing bonk on the ramps of the Alpe d'Huez. Fortunately, his teammate Richie Porte was able to bail him out with an energy gel and a wheel to follow, and, despite incurring a 20-second penalty for an illegal feed, his Tour was saved.

Going back to your sportive and your own private low blood sugar hell, how did it happen? When you're riding a long event such as a sportive, your body is drawing fuel from two main sources. The first, when you're riding at lower intensities, is your fat reserves, a huge potential reservoir of fuel. The second, carbohydrates, fuelling harder efforts, is provided by your body's stored supply in your muscles and liver in the form of glycogen, giving about 90 minutes of energy, and the fuel you're providing as you eat and drink on the bike. These two energy sources are not discrete of one another and, depending on how hard you're riding, you'll draw from somewhere along a fat and carbohydrate continuum. However, above a certain intensity, usually somewhere in mid to upper Zone 2 for most riders, is a point where the body does switch over fully to carbohydrates. Slightly lower than this point, sometimes referred to as 'fat max', is another key cut-off. This is the intensity at which energy from fat utilisation and the carbohydrates that you're able to take on and process combine to preserve that 90-minute reservoir of stored energy. If you consistently ride above this intensity, you'll create an energy overdraft and slowly start chipping away at that limited store. You might get away with this for a few hours but eventually that energy store will be totally depleted and then you're 100 per cent reliant on the carbohydrates you can supply and your fat reserves. You can only take on and utilise a limited amount of carbohydrates and certainly not enough to fuel riding on its own. As we've already discussed, you have plenty of energy stored as fat, even if you're super lean, but that's only useful if you're riding super steady.

So, despite seemingly fuelling well, you pushed a fraction too hard earlier on during the ride and now, on the final climb, you're paying the price. You felt fine on the flat run in to the climb as you were sitting in the wheels and able to utilise your fat reserves but as you start climbing, your muscles demand carbohydrates. You have a small amount in your bloodstream from the fuel you took on 30 minutes or so ago but that won't last long; the gel you've just taken is sitting in your stomach and your body's carbohydrate stores were run dry kilometres back. Without carbohydrates to fuel the Zone 3/4 climbing effort, your muscles stop working and, with the brain totally reliant on carbohydrates, the characteristic light-headed and dizzy sensations of a full-on bonk soon follow. A gel or a generous swig of sports drink or soda in your mouth might give a momentary boost or, if you have low enough gears, you might be able to crawl over the top of the climb but, either way, it's not going to be pretty.

It's a fine line and fuelling endurance activity is always a nutritional knife edge. You can certainly give yourself a bit more wriggle room by developing your ability to utilise fat as a fuel but, in the end, it comes down to strict discipline regarding both pacing and fuelling. Learn what you're capable of in training and don't expect some miraculous event-day boost. You probably won't have a Richie Porte in tow to bail you out.

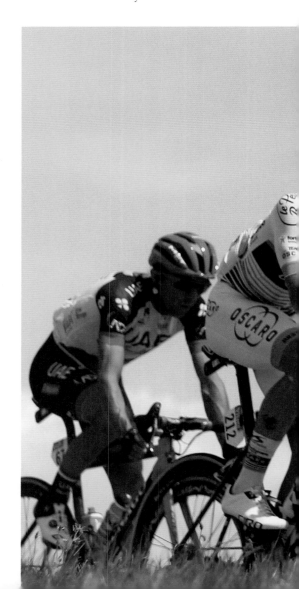

▼ Having a bonk probably happens to all riders at some point but, with good pacing and fuelling, can be avoided.

It's important that your training rides mimic not only the terrain of your target events as closely as possible but also how you intend to ride them. The café stop is a prime example of this and unfortunately this enjoyable tradition is responsible for many riders bonking on event day. That 20–30-minute sit down, caffeine boost and slice of sugar-filled cake gives your body a chance to reboot. You'll digest some of the food sitting in your stomach, raise your blood sugar level and even replace some of your body's carbohydrate stores. This means it allows you to ride unrealistically hard pre- and post-café stop but get away with it. Physiologically, a 5-hour ride without a significant break is very different to a 5-hour ride broken up with a 30-minute café stop. If you try to ride them both at the same intensity, you're likely to come unstuck. So, if you're training for a long event and are aiming to complete it effectively non-stop, a significant number of your training rides should reflect this and you'll have to forego the café stop. If this is unthinkable for you, you'll either have to factor in a similar break during your event or adjust your pacing strategy accordingly and ride more conservatively.

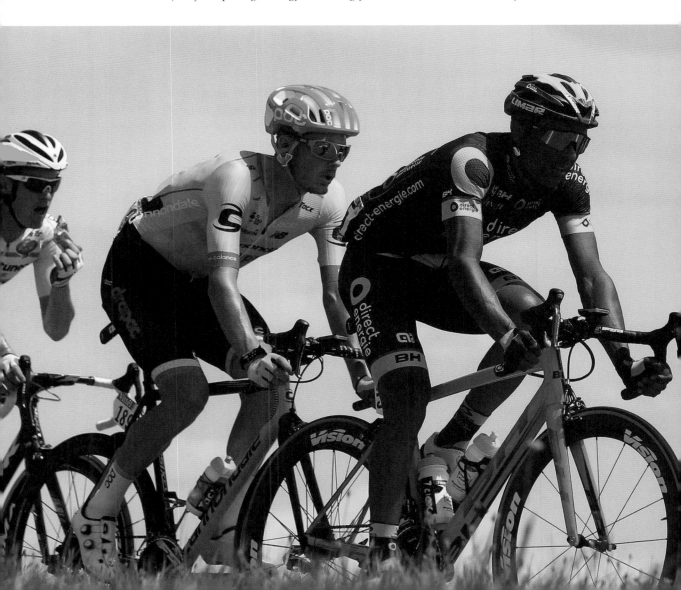

Weight loss

One of the biggest areas of potential gain for a huge number of cyclists is shedding some excess fat. It's not glamorous, it's hard and it's definitely not as instantly gratifying as a new set of wheels, but it's practically guaranteed to make you faster. Numerous studies have been performed showing just how much weight affects riding speed, especially when climbing. Typically, for a rider on a 5km (3 mile) 8 per cent grade climb, every 2.5kg (5½lb) of extra weight would cost 30–40 seconds.

Obviously, though, if you're also training, along with losing weight you're likely to see a bump in your FTP. Combine this with some weight loss and the argument for skipping that extra serving of dessert becomes even more compelling. Let's assume that our rider is able to hold 250 watts for the climb. As we've already seen, through losing 2.5kg alone, he'll save 30–40 seconds. If he doesn't skip desserts but his training gives him an extra 10 watts, he's looking at a saving of 40 seconds and 20 watts would give him 85 seconds. Now, if he manages to shed 2.5kg and gain 20 watts, he's looking at a KOM-smashing saving of over 2 minutes.

Power to weight

This combination of sustainable power and weight gives one of the most important metrics for predicting cycling performance, especially when the road kicks uphill: power to weight ratio. Expressed as w/kg, your power to weight at threshold (FTP) is a key statistic to track. If we take our example rider again and assume he was climbing near to his FTP, for his power to weight ratio we'd simply take his output, 250 watts, and divide it by his weight, 75kg (165lb), to give a power to weight at threshold ratio of 3.33w/kg. If he managed his 2.5kg weight loss and 20 watt gain, this would rise to 3.88w/kg. There are a number of tables available online that show what this figure means in comparison to other riders and, for our guy, his 3.72w/kg would place him on a par with a typical Cat 3 racer. To put things in a perspective, a world class professional rider would have a power to weight ratio at threshold over 6w/kg so, at 75kg, possessing an FTP of 450 watts.

Although weight loss will have the greatest impact on your climbing ability, it'll also have benefits for other areas of your riding. You'll reduce your frontal profile

'Analyse the amount of energy you need, find your metabolic rate but avoid going too far under this requirement. You'll obviously lose weight if you're below it but it'll also have a negative effect on your performance. When you're training hard isn't the best time to try and lose weight. We'll also look at the riders' body composition, not just their weight on the scales, as we don't want them losing muscle mass.'

JULIA SCHULZE, TEAM DOCTOR, CANYON/SRAM

and, especially if you lose some bulk around your midriff, be able to hold a more aerodynamic position and be faster on the flat. Off the mark, you'll have less mass to move, so whether it's leaving the gate on the track or punching away from a slow hairpin in a criterium, you'll be faster.

There is a point for all riders, particularly if you start losing significant muscle mass, where weight loss can cause you to start losing power. However, as long as your approach to weight loss is sensible, it's highly unlikely that this will be a concern.

Weight loss tips

Having established that losing some weight is likely to improve your cycling, how do you go about it? Despite what many diet plans and quack nutritionists would have you believe, there's no real secret to successful weight loss. It's as simple and boring as discipline, time and sensible healthy eating.

FIND YOUR COMPOSITION

It's important to think in terms of fat loss rather than weight loss as, unless you're carrying excessive upper body muscle mass, you're ideally wanting to preserve your lean mass and lose excess fat. Despite what the adage says, the scales do lie. If you think that you can afford to lose a few pounds but are unsure what target to set yourself, the best thing to do is to find out your body composition. There are a number of ways of doing this, from high-tech body analysis pods to humble skin-fold calipers, but all will give you an idea of how much of your weight comprises lean tissue and how much is fat. Although appearing to be fairly low-tech and crude, skin-fold calipers, used by an experienced professional, are probably the most accessible and reliable method, and are still used by the majority of professional cycling teams. A well-qualified personal trainer at your local gym should be able to conduct a skin-fold test and, as long as the same PT performs subsequent tests, it's probably the best way to track your body composition. Avoid scales and handheld devices that claim to measure body composition using bio-impedance, passing a small electrical current through your body, as the results they give vary massively depending on hydration level and a number of other factors.

TRACK CALORIES IN AND CALORIES OUT

Keeping a food diary serves two purposes that both facilitate fat loss. It firstly forces you to be aware of what you're eating and less likely to mindlessly eat that biscuit or slice of cake. Secondly, especially if you use an online app, it allows you to track your calorie intake and calculate a daily target calorie goal, including an estimate of your basal metabolic rate based on age and weight, that will allow you to reach your fat loss goal. Be aware that the estimated metabolic rate, although a good starting point, is only an estimate and, as you monitor your fat loss, you may have to adapt it. Similarly, when calculating the calories you're burning through exercise, estimates from heart rate and so on are notoriously inaccurate and, although using a power meter considerably increases accuracy, it's still not 100 per cent.

As a general rule, a safe and manageable rate of fat loss is approximately 0.5kg (1lb) per week. To achieve this, you need a net calorie deficit of 3,500 calories per week or 500 calories per day. By using a calorie tracker and keeping an eye on how your body composition/weight changes, you'll be able to adjust the figures to your own physiology and needs.

As with training, though, more isn't necessarily more. Don't try and consistently exceed a deficit of 500 calories as you'll significantly compromise your ability to train and, by putting your body into a starvation response, risk losing valuable lean tissue rather than fat.

RIDING ISN'T A REASON TO EAT WHAT YOU WANT

A mistake a lot of riders make is that they think, as they're putting in the miles, it gives them carte blanche to eat whatever they want. Unfortunately, if you're wanting to lose some fat, exercise alone just doesn't cut it and you have to apply some discipline to your diet. When you look at the volume of riding that full time professionals put in and they're still having to be super diligent with their diet, you definitely can't just eat what you want.

One kilogram (2.2lb) of body fat is worth about 7,000 calories so, to lose a kilogram, you need to achieve this energy deficit. From a cycling point of view, if you're out riding at Zone 2 endurance intensity, you'll burn approximately 600 calories/hr and would therefore require just under 12 hours. This obviously doesn't take into account the fuel you consume while riding, so to lose fat from exercise alone takes an awful lot of work.

LOSE WEIGHT DURING THE OFF SEASON

The best time to try to lose some fat is during the off season, when training intensity is at its lowest. During this time of year, your sessions will generally be steadier and less performance orientated. This means you can probably get away with slightly less fuel and running a bigger calorie deficit. Once you start ramping up the intensity of your training, you won't be able to perform the sessions optimally and recover adequately unless you're fully fuelling.

HARVEST LOW-HANGING FRUIT

Cutting out alcohol and processed food, especially refined sugar, are two of the easiest ways to reduce your calorie intake. Regarding sugar, if you regularly drink soda, a 330ml can contains 140 calories, so just a few of those a day and you're wiping out your 500-calorie deficit. If you can, avoid switching to artificially sweetened alternatives as it's been shown that artificial sweeteners increase the body's desire to consume sugar. Don't forget, though, sugar is a great fuel for exercise and, although you should be looking to minimise it in your day-to-day diet, when you're on the bike, it's perfectly acceptable.

FUEL THE SESSION

We've already discussed the importance of this earlier on in the chapter but it applies equally here. You won't be able to perform a high-intensity interval session if you're under-fuelled or restricting carbohydrate intake. Equally, on a rest day, do you really

▶ There's no doubt being lighter can make you faster but not if the weight loss costs you power or training quality.

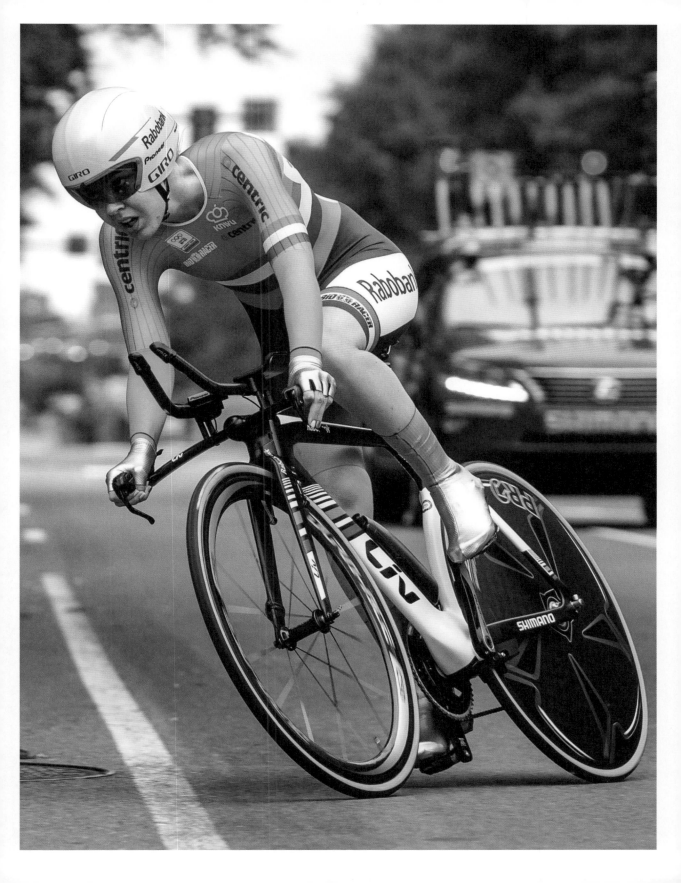

need that big bowl of porridge? On a long ride day, you might be well over the target 500 calories deficit and struggling to eat enough calories to bring yourself up to it, but it's important you do or you risk sacrificing lean tissue. Conversely, if you're having a rest day, the food you're allowed can seem meagre. It's important, whether you're trying to lose fat or not, that you tailor your diet to the training you're doing and don't just eat the same, day in, day out.

PRIORITISE PROTEIN

Maintenance of your lean tissue mass is a priority and the nutrient that facilities that, especially during periods when you're trying to lose fat, is protein. Depending on your training, you can cut back on carbohydrates but you can't afford to skimp on quality protein. Maintaining your protein intake also has the benefit of helping you to feel full.

A male cyclist will typically require 1.2–1.6g/kg/day of protein, with female riders requiring about 15 per cent less (1.0–1.4g/kg/day). For an 80kg (176lb) male cyclist, this translates to 96–128g (3½–4½oz) of protein, which could be provided by:

3-egg omelette	= 18g
Pistachios, handful 25g	= 5g
Tuna sandwich, 1 can (drained)	= 27g
Cottage cheese, half cup 80g	= 18g
2 turkey breast steaks 120g	= 43g
500ml (18fl oz) whole milk	= 16g
Total	**= 127g**

A 60kg (132lb) female cyclist would need 54–72g (2–2½oz) of protein, which could be provided by:

2-egg omelette	= 12g
Pistachios, handful 25g	= 5g
Tuna sandwich, ½ can (drained)	= 13.5g
Cottage cheese, quarter cup 40g	= 9g
1 turkey breast steak 60g	= 21.5g
250ml (9fl oz) whole milk	= 8g
Total	**= 69g**

Vegetarian and vegan cyclists need to be particularly careful that they're consuming adequate protein and that it contains the full range of essential amino acids.

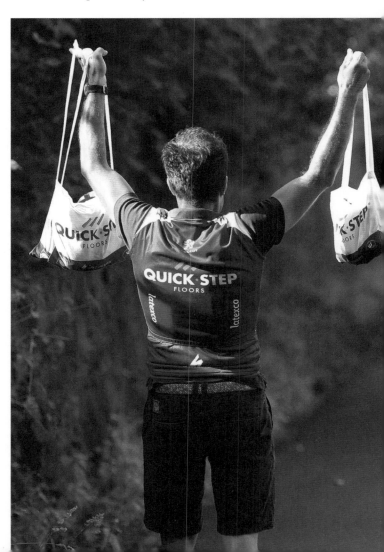

▼ When you're training or racing hard isn't the time to try and lose weight. You've got to fuel your engine.

'First and foremost, you should exist as a healthy person and eat appropriately. Don't try to cut calories drastically or to crash weight off, effective fat loss is a gradual process. At no point should you feel ravenously hungry because all that does is make your body store fat more and it backfires on you, and I've experienced that. I had a nutritionist who'd test my body composition with calipers and, when I was trying to lose weight too aggressively by dramatically cutting calories and skipping meals, yes, the scales would go down but only because I'd lost muscle and gained fat. He'd say, congratulations, you've made yourself slower and reduced the effectiveness of your last block of training by not having enough fuel.'

PHIL GAIMON, EX-PRO WITH GARMIN-SHARP AND CANNONDALE-DRAPAC

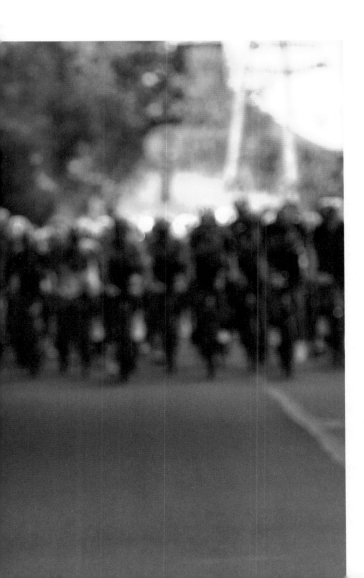

AVOID FADDY DIETS

Whether it's by cutting out a particular food group, fasting on a given day or not eating after a certain time of day, all diets 'work' by making it more difficult to eat normally and therefore creating a net calorie deficit. Don't buy into the hype of faddy diets – it's far better and more effective in the long term to make sustainable small changes to how you eat. Certainly, any diet that promises fast or crash weight loss will not be suitable if you're also wanting to maintain structured and effective training. Also, steer clear of processed 'low-fat' food as it's likely to be loaded with sugar.

DON'T PUT IT ON

Although carrying a few extra pounds during the winter can be useful for keeping warm and avoiding getting ill, try to limit any off-season weight gain. Having to crash weight off in the pre-season in an attempt to get in race shape is not going to be complementary to the increase in training intensity at that time of year. Give yourself a bit more freedom during the off season but keep tabs on things and don't let any weight gain get out of hand.

Hydration

Hydration for endurance sport has been an area of intense debate recently. On one side of the argument are researchers who claim that drinking to thirst is plenty enough and trying to hydrate beyond this is potentially dangerous, risking hyponatremia or 'water poisoning'. On the other side is the sports drink industry, quoting studies that claim that as little as a 2 per cent drop in body weight due to sweating (1.6kg/3½lb for an 80kg/176lb rider) will impair performance noticeably, 4 per cent will decrease your capacity for muscular work and, at 5 per cent, heat exhaustion can become an issue and your capacity for work will drop by up to 30 per cent. More confusion has also been added by professional cycling teams talking about the use of functional dehydration, purposely allowing their riders to dehydrate by 4 per cent, to enhance their power to weight ratio and therefore improve climbing performance. As with most things, the truth is somewhere in the middle and maintaining hydration while cycling is actually fairly simple, uncomplicated and intuitive.

Off the bike

If you're regularly monitoring your weight, any sudden or unexpected drops are likely to indicate that you're dehydrated. On Grand Tours, teams will weigh riders daily to check hydration levels. Keep an eye on the colour of your urine. Refer to the chart on

▼ Don't be confused by extreme viewpoints, hydration for endurance sports isn't a case of all or nothing but a sensible middle ground.

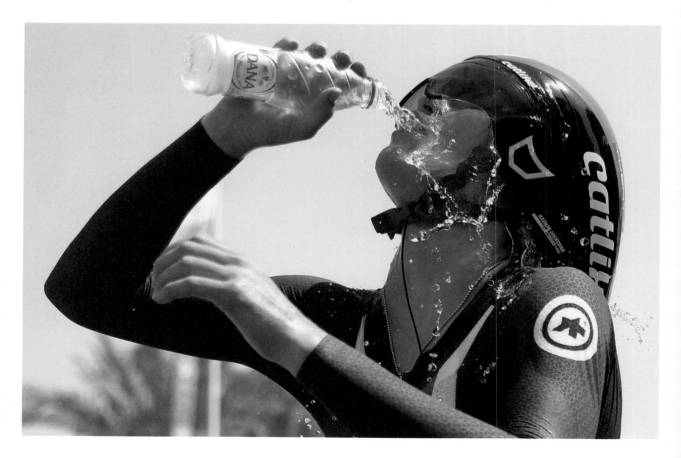

CRAMP

For such a common occurrence, it's surprising that the exact reason and mechanisms behind cramping are still largely unknown. If you have ever suffered cramp during a long training ride, sportive or race, you, like many others, probably pointed the finger at the heat, poor hydration and a lack of electrolyte intake. However, recent work with Ironman triathletes, racing in extreme heat in Kona at the World Championships, found no link at all, and although some studies have shown that consuming a 6 per cent carbohydrate sports drink can help prevent cramp, other studies have failed to back this up. A sudden increase in exercise intensity is a factor, so if you suddenly ride harder or longer than you're used to, you can expect to cramp. However, this doesn't explain night cramps. Some studies of long-term sufferers of cramp have shown magnesium supplementation to be helpful. Anecdotal evidence suggests that stretching can also help to alleviate cramp and that regular stretching can help prevent cramp in muscles that are prone to it or that have previously been injured.

If you suffered from cramp during an event, when it hadn't been an issue in training, the most likely explanation is that you simply pushed a bit harder or further than your body was used to. You should always keep on top of your electrolyte and fluid intake, and regular mobility work should be a must for all riders, but your cramping is probably due to poor pacing or inadequate training.

page 164 that shows the colour you should be looking to maintain, but it's basically pale straw. Along with monitoring your hydration level, try to drink 2–3 litres (3½–5¼ pints) of fluids a day, whether you're riding or not. Fruit and vegetable juices, sports drinks and water all count towards this target but alcohol, tea, coffee and sugar-laden soft drinks don't.

On the bike

As with eating to fuel the particular ride you're doing, the same applies to hydration. For rides under 60 minutes, plain water is fine. For longer rides, it makes sense to combine drinking with calorie intake – 500ml (18fl oz) of typical sports drink mixed at 4–6 per cent (4–6g of carbohydrate per 100ml/3 ½fl oz of water) will give you 20–24g (around ¾oz) of carbohydrate. Different brands of sports drinks use varying blends of sugars and carbohydrate sources. Cheaper products will use primarily sucrose. More expensive brands blend fructose and maltodextrin, a long-chain carbohydrate, to provide a more staggered release, and tend to be easier on your stomach. Experiment to find a brand that encourages you to drink and sits well in your stomach. A sports drink will also deliver the electrolytes your body needs to function properly. Incidentally, it's by diluting the electrolytes in your body by drinking excessive amounts of plain water that, in extreme cases, hyponatremia or 'water poisoning' can occur. As long as the fluid you're taking on contains electrolytes to replace the ones you're losing in sweat, this can't occur. Remember, there will also be electrolytes in the food you're consuming.

If you stick to plain water, you're missing out on an easy way to get energy into your system; it won't stimulate you to drink in the same way as a sports drink and it can sit in your stomach and leave you feeling bloated. A good budget option is a 50/50 mix of pineapple juice and water with a pinch of salt added.

Although it is possible to conduct a sweat test to calculate your fluid requirements, where you weigh yourself before and after riding to work out fluid loss, I've never found this to be necessary. There are so many variables to take into account that it's just not worth the effort. Working on having a sip from my bottle every 10–15 minutes from the start of the ride seems to work well and, depending on the temperature, my body seems to do a good job of regulating the size of the sip and results in a fluid intake of 500–750ml (18–26fl oz) per hour.

As long as you take small and regular sips from the start and, if you're on a long ride, drink a 4–6 per cent carbohydrate sports drink containing electrolytes, you're not going to go far wrong.

Once you get back from a ride, rehydration does play an important role in the recovery process. You don't need to go mad, though, and you'll be starting the rehydration process with your protein recovery drink. Again, just keep drinking regularly in the hours following your ride and monitor your urine colour.

URINE COLOUR CHART

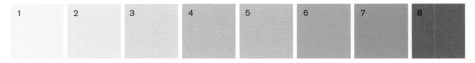

Urine colour charts are simple tools to help you to assess hydration level. You should aim to have urine in the 1–3 bands. If your urine is darker (4–8), this would suggest you need to drink more fluid.

Be aware that some multivitamin supplements can affect the colour of your urine, reducing the validity of this chart. In this case you should consider other methods of monitoring hydration.

Supplements: no magic bullets

Although there are certain legal substances, such as caffeine, sodium bicarbonate, beta alanine, nitrates and creatine, that have been proven to increase cycling performance, the boost they'll give is definitely in the marginal gains category. There are far more significant gains to be made first, with your training, regular nutrition, technique and kit, before exploring supplementation.

However, there are two supplements that, as endurance athletes, you should consider taking. They're not going to supercharge your cycling but they will make you healthier and more able to absorb and adapt to your training load.

The first is a quality fish oil containing the omega-3 fatty acid eicosapentaenoic acid (EPA). Used extensively by professional riders, it gives a number of benefits. Omega-3 fats are not only linked to reduced inflammation but also to positively influencing blood vessels and protein synthesis. This means that, in times of heavy training, they can help in the maintenance of muscle mass. Although it's possible to obtain omega-3 from oily fish and seeds, it's the ratio with omega-6 that's key. Omega-6 is very prevalent in modern diets and, to ensure the optimal 1:1 ratio, supplementation of omega-3 is often necessary. You should aim to obtain 2g of EPA daily, which, using a high-dose omega-3 product, will equate to 3–5 capsules. Unfortunately, cheaper cod liver oil just doesn't contain the levels of EPA necessary so it's important to buy a quality product.

The second, for riders living in the Northern Hemisphere and from September through to late March, is Vitamin D. During the winter months, low light levels result in reduced synthesis of Vitamin D in our bodies. Even if you do manage to get out each day, winter daylight isn't intense enough to stimulate production. This can lead to poor bone health, suppressed immunity, reduced recovery and increased fatigue. Although it is possible to obtain Vitamin D from your food (oily fish are especially rich), it's now recommended by health authorities that adults should take a daily supplement of 10 μg.

Beating doping

In 2017, the UK magazine *Cycling Weekly* anonymously surveyed its readers and found that 5 per cent of those who responded admitted to doping. There have also been a number of cases of riders in time trials, taking part in Masters events and at Gran Fondos testing positive for banned substances. Unfortunately, most anti-doping resources are devoted to the top levels of sport so, to a certain degree, below the top tier, a self-policing approach is necessary. Most national governing bodies and anti-doping agencies can be contacted directly and allow for suspicious behaviour to be anonymously reported. There are a number of things you should be on the lookout for, and these include:

- Coaches or riders discussing doping or doping methods.
- A rider showing a sudden improvement in their performances and results.
- Someone handling a suspicious package.
- A rider regularly dropping out before the finish of races to avoid testing.
- A rider or coach offering you a supplement you've never heard of.

Obviously, this list isn't exhaustive and, if you do have any suspicions, you should report them with as much detail as possible. It's up to us as riders to protect our sport and to ensure we're competing on a level playing field.

The amount of testing being carried out at all levels of the sport is increasing, though, and in the UK, for example, whether you are competing in your local club 10-mile time trial, a local circuit race or even riding a sportive, as a British Cycling member you could be tested. As the national federation of cycling in Great Britain,

British Cycling adopts UKAD Rules. This means that all British Cycling members agree to adhere to these rules. Most other national governing bodies operate similar policies. Part of this means members agree to being tested at any time in any location in and out of competition. So, in theory, the testers could come knocking at your door anytime if you're a member of your national governing body.

The higher the level of competition, the more likely you are to be tested. For National level events, there are no hard and fast rules about who will be tested, from the winner to the last rider home – anyone could be tested. For World Masters events, if you set a world record, for it to be ratified you will be tested. Winners, second place riders and a number of randomly selected athletes are also commonly tested.

It's your responsibility as a rider to ensure that you're not unwittingly taking any substances that might lead you to be found guilty of an Anti-Doping Rule Violation (ADRV). You should be aware of the Prohibited List, an International Standard identifying substances and methods prohibited in sport, both in and out of competition. The Prohibited List is updated at least annually, following an extensive consultation process with stakeholders facilitated by WADA's List Expert Group. An updated list comes into effect on 1 January of each year, and in accordance with the Code is generally published three months before implementation. To find the most up to date Prohibited List, consult the WADA website: www.wada-ama.org.

Over-the-counter medication presents a risk for all athletes, and a product that may contain no banned substances in one country can have significantly different ingredients if purchased in another. The Global Drug Reference Online (Global DRO) allows you to check any over-the-counter medication: www.globaldro.com/Home.

Along with over-the-counter medication, supplements probably carry the greatest risk for being found guilty of an ADRV. The main problem is contamination of an apparently clean product with a banned substance. This can happen surprisingly easily. For example, if a manufacturer produces both body-building and cycling supplements in the same factory, there can easily be ingredients in the body-building products that, although not banned in the sport of body-building, are banned substances for cyclists. In such a situation, it's easy to see how contamination could take place. More sinister are manufacturers who spike their products with known but banned performance enhancers to raise their effectiveness and marketability.

Unfortunately, if you unknowingly take such a contaminated supplement and it causes you to be found guilty of an ADRV, ignorance is no defence. This is the principle of strict liability, where riders are solely responsible for any prohibited substance found in their system, whether there was an intention to cheat or not.

If you do decide to take a supplement, you can minimise but not eliminate the risk by checking whether the product is on the Informed-Sport website www.informed-sport.com. Batches of products that carry this logo have been independently tested and those batches are listed on the site. Informed-Sport is a risk-minimisation programme; it does not remove risk entirely. If a rider has made a decision to use a supplement, they can reduce the risk by taking a supplement that has been subjected to credible testing and appropriate manufacturing controls, rather than none at all.

▶ As athletes we're responsible for what goes into our bodies and for helping to keep our sport clean.

How to improve your cycling performance

Fuel your training

Your nutrition, both on and off the bike, should be dictated by the training you're doing. Intense training will necessitate readily available carbohydrates such as gels, whereas slower-paced riding can be fuelled with 'real' food. Don't eat the same meals every day – for example, if you're on a rest day, you don't need a big bowl of porridge for breakfast.

Pacing! Pacing! Pacing!

If you're suffering from digestive distress on the bike but you're not eating unsuitable foods, it's almost certainly down to poor pacing. Pacing and fuelling are intrinsically linked and if you're pushing too hard, your digestive system will shut down. Practise your pacing and fuelling in training and make sure you stick to your tried and tested approach during any events.

Cut out the café stop

Not on every ride, but if you're intending to complete a long event non-stop, you have to practise this in training. A 5-hour ride with a 20–30-minute stop for coffee and cake is significantly different physiologically to a straight-through 5-hour ride and can give you a false impression of the pace you'd be able to maintain.

Shed some fat

A large majority of riders would benefit from shedding a bit of excess fat and not just when climbing. The best time to try to lose fat is when you're not training hard and can maintain a negative calorie balance without it compromising the effectiveness of your sessions. Sustainable changes to your diet will always be more effective in the long term than faddy diets, and fat loss should be steady and sensible.

Keep hydration simple

Don't be bamboozled by all of the controversy surrounding hydration in endurance sport. Monitor your weight and urine colour to check day-to-day hydration. Plain water or squash is fine for rides under 60 minutes. For longer rides, opt for a 4–6 per cent sports drink containing electrolytes, have a sip every 10–15 minutes, and look to drink 500–750ml (18–26fl oz) per hour.

Be suspicious of supplements

If you've ticked every box in this book regarding optimising your kit, training and regular nutrition, certain supplements might give you a very small additional edge. However, there are no legal magic bullets and it's possible to waste a lot of money on almost immeasurable gains.

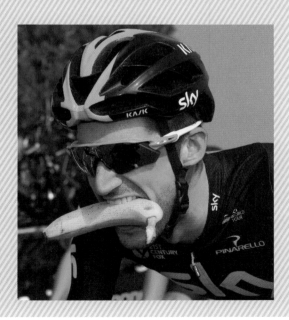

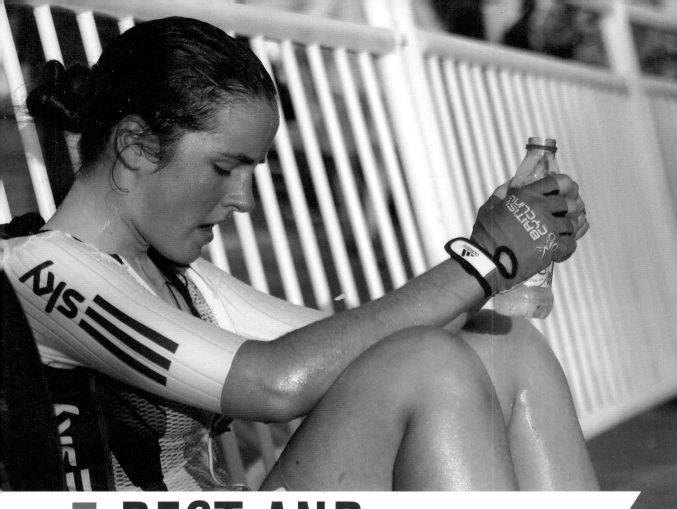

7 REST AND RECOVERY

ALONG WITH SCHEDULING IN ADEQUATE REST DAYS AND EASIER RECOVERY WEEKS IN YOUR TRAINING PLAN, THERE ARE A NUMBER OF PRACTICAL STEPS YOU CAN TAKE TO MAXIMISE YOUR RECOVERY FROM TRAINING AND, IN DOING SO, MAKE GREATER GAINS FROM IT.

RESTING HEART RATE

Getting into the habit of checking your pulse first thing in the morning is an excellent way of getting a heads-up for the early warning signs of non-functional overreaching or a looming illness. Once you've got over the shock of your alarm going off, lie back and relax for a minute and find your radial (wrist) pulse. Count the beats in a minute and note it down in your training log. You can just count for 30 or even 15 seconds and multiply by 2 and 4 respectively, but a full minute gives a more accurate reading. After a week or so, you should get a good idea of what your typical resting heart rate is. As your training progresses, expect to see your resting pulse steadily dropping. However, if you notice an increase or decrease in rate from one day to another of more than five beats per minute, take a rest day or only train very lightly.

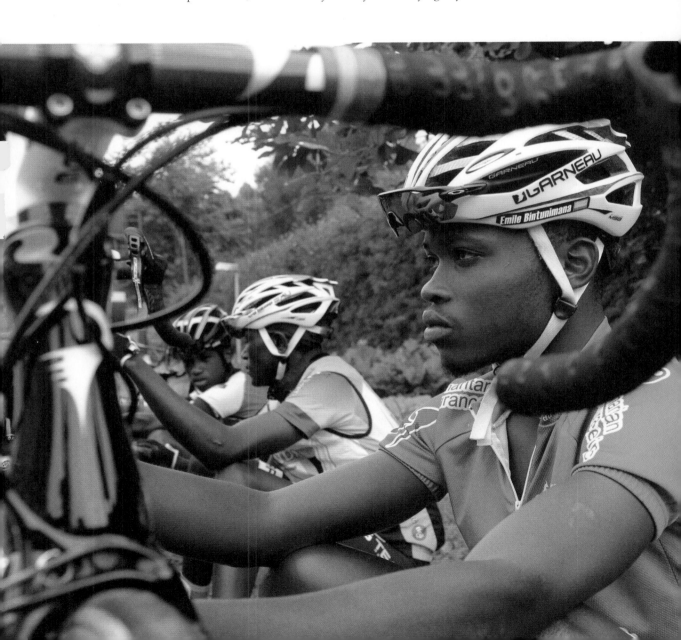

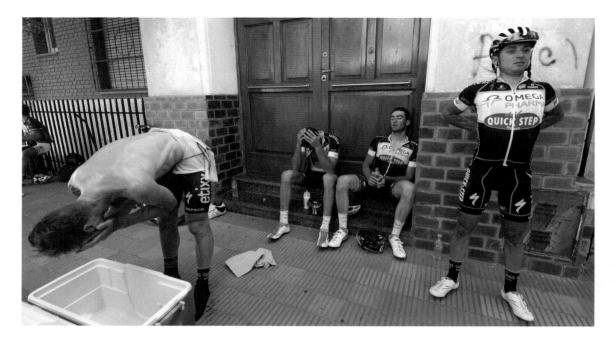

RAPID WEIGHT LOSS

For many riders, losing a bit of excess fat can be one of the biggest bonuses of following a structured training plan, but too rapid weight loss is a sign of non-functional overreaching combined with under-fuelling and indicates that you might be losing muscle tissue as well as fat. Daily weigh-ins and plotting your weight on a graph is the best way to monitor your weight. Make sure you weigh at the same time each day. Expect to see daily fluctuations of up to or even over a kilogram (2.2lbs), but if the overall trend shows weight loss of much more than 1kg from one week to the next, it's not necessarily a good thing. Obviously, some people have more fat to lose initially than others and can expect to see more rapid weight loss but any sudden significant increases in weight loss should be viewed with suspicion.

POOR SLEEP

With the saddle time you'll be logging, you will probably sleep better than you've ever slept, but having problems sleeping is one of the classic signs of non-functional overreaching. As sleep is when your body repairs itself and recovers, not sleeping throws you into a vicious circle. Typically, an athlete who's in a state of non-functional overreaching has problems getting to sleep, complaining of restless legs or just feeling wide awake. As well as maybe backing off your training for a couple of days, look at your bedtime routine and sleeping environment. If possible, avoid training within two hours of going to bed or, if you have to train late, factor in a relaxing mobility session when you get in, followed by a hot bath and maybe some meditation or mindfulness work. Drink some hot milk, but avoid tea or coffee any later than midday. Avoid watching television or going on the computer in the bedroom or immediately before going to bed. Make sure your bedroom is quiet, genuinely dark and not too warm. If you are struggling to sleep, don't lay there stressing and clock-watching. Get up, make yourself some warm milk, read for half an hour and then try going back to bed.

EXCESSIVE MUSCLE SORENESS

DOMS (delayed onset muscle soreness) is characterised by soreness in your muscles 48–72 hours after exercise. It's part of the normal inflammation and adaptation process associated with training, is perfectly normal and is part of how muscles become stronger. Over 24 hours the soreness normally fades and recovery techniques can speed up this process. If you're consistently overdoing it, though, the soreness will not ease and your legs will feel continuously sore, heavy and tired.

IRRITABILITY AND POOR MOOD

Exercise should improve your mood and give you a genuine mental lift. As well as the very real 'exercise high' elicited by chemicals released in your brain during exercise, sticking to a regular training plan will improve feelings of self-worth and give a genuine sense of achievement. However, too much training, combined with not enough recovery and insufficient sleep, can really bring you down. As well as feeling irritable, snappy or a bit low, one of the classic signs of non-functional overreaching is genuinely starting to dread training sessions. We all have days when getting out to train is a real effort but, in the main, you should look forward to it.

If a state of non-functional overreaching is ignored, not only will you be failing to get the most out of the effort you're putting in on the bike, you also risk making yourself extremely ill. Overtraining syndrome is a medical condition, requiring a medical diagnosis, and describes a prolonged maladaptation, the result of a continued too-high training load and too little recovery. This condition is extremely serious and if you think you're at risk, you should consult with a qualified medical professional.

'It's all about overcoming that "more is more" athletes' mentality and realising that a day off can be as beneficial as another day of training. There's obviously a volume of training that you have to do and it's normal to feel a certain amount of tiredness but, more and more, the emphasis is on quality rather than quantity. For me, the real warning sign is deeper fatigue. I constantly feel tired, I have no energy when I wake up and I don't have the motivation to get out on the bike. When I am on the bike, I just can't produce the power or push my heart rate as high as I know it should go during a particular effort. That's when I know I've got to listen to my body and back off. I've got so much better at taking my recovery seriously.' **TIFFANY CROMWELL**, CANYON/SRAM

If you find yourself exhibiting more than two or three of the signs described for more than a couple of consecutive days, you should take action. Give yourself an extra rest day and possibly schedule in a recovery week. Take a look at your training over the preceding weeks. What have you changed? Have you ramped up either intensity or volume too quickly and have you been taking regular rest days and recovery weeks? Equally, look at your non-cycling life. Has work been especially busy or stressful? Has your baby not been sleeping through the night? Remember, these non-cycling factors have to be included in your 'training load' and can't just be ignored. Go back to the basic template of the three essential sessions, two quality midweek workouts and a longer weekend ride, stick with just that for a few weeks and, if you find that the signs of non-functional overreaching diminish, incrementally add some more volume. However, remember the golden rule that quality always trumps quantity and that three workouts consistently done well are always better than five or six compromised sessions. Along with trying to incorporate some of the recovery techniques described later in the chapter, take practical steps to increase the time you have available for recovery. For example, if you're normally out for 4 hours on your weekend ride and include a significant café break, lose the café stop and ride for a solid 3 hours instead. Use the extra hour you've got back for a dedicated off your feet post-ride chill-out and maybe even a nap.

Enhancing your recovery

Along with ensuring that you schedule in the appropriate amount of recovery time for the training you're doing, there are a number of techniques you can use to enhance your recovery.

COOLING DOWN

In Chapter 4 we talked about the importance of warming up and cooling down. Always try to spend the final 10–15 minutes of every ride spinning a low gear in Zone 1. This can take a fair bit of discipline if you're trying to nudge up your average speed or power for the ride, get sucked into an end-of-ride sprint or are pressed for time, but it really does make a difference to the recovery process. It's a common occurrence on Grand Tours these days for the presentations to be delayed because the GC leader is completing their cool-down. You should view your cool-down both as the end of your current ride and the start of your next one.

NUTRITION

Following the guidelines in Chapter 6 regarding post-ride nutrition will definitely aid the recovery process. Prioritise protein and consider supplementing with a quality fish oil product. It's not just about post-ride nutrition, though – if you fuel poorly during the ride and allow yourself to become dehydrated or too depleted, this will have a knock-on effect on your recovery and future rides. For hard interval workouts,

▶ There are a number of practical steps you can take to optimise your post-ride recovery.

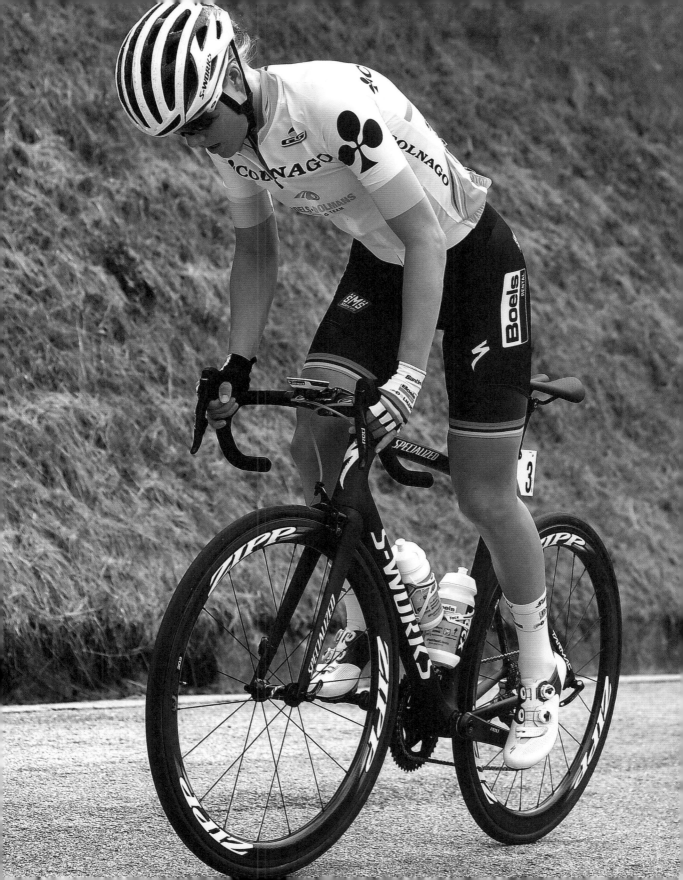

a good idea can be to have a second bottle on the bike containing a protein recovery drink or, for longer rides with efforts, a sachet that you can mix with some water. You should aim to have this bottle during the final 10–20 minutes of the ride, when you're cooling down. This ensures that you're kick-starting your recovery and starting your preparation for your next ride.

GET OFF YOUR FEET

Follow the pros' lead and aim to spend at least some time horizontal post-ride. You'd be staggered just how lazy elite athletes are when not training and how seriously they devote themselves to doing nothing and keeping their weight off their feet.

> 'I've been retired for about a year and I still won't stand up. I was a Halloween party last night and we're all standing in someone's living room at a bar and I'm desperately looking for a stool. It's burned deep into me that you don't stand up, you never stand up. You lean or you sit and if you can you lie down. I wonder how many years I'll be done racing before that mentality goes away?'
> PHIL GAIMON EX-PRO WITH GARMIN-SHARP AND CANNONDALE-DRAPAC

▼ Mobilisation, massage or just getting off your feet can all help you recover from a ride.

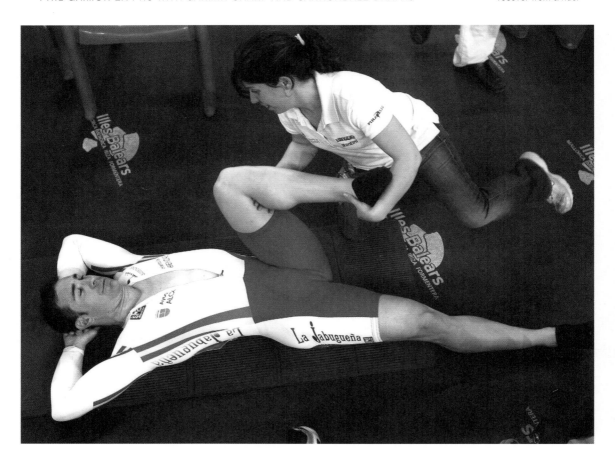

It can be hard if you have a family and have already been out riding for 4 hours or more on a weekend, but do try. It doesn't have to be hours on the sofa. Grab a pillow for your head and lie on the floor with your backside close to a wall and your legs elevated. Shuffle closer to the wall, keep your legs straight but soft at the knees and you should feel a gentle stretch on your hamstrings. Chill in this position for 5 minutes for every hour you've just ridden. It feels great, aids venous return, and gently stretches and relaxes your lower back and hamstrings.

MOBILISE

If you have the time post-ride once you've showered and eaten, working through some of the exercises in the mobility routine described in Chapter 5 will aid recovery. You can view the TASMT, using a foam roller and a trigger ball, as a poor man's massage.

MASSAGE

Although viewed as an essential part of any pro cyclist's routine, the actual physiological benefits of massage are far from proven. It definitely doesn't flush lactic acid, as is often claimed, and the gains are probably as much down to relaxation and a psychological boost as anything else. However, that doesn't mean that a massage is a waste of time.

If you're not on a pro team, daily or even weekly massages probably aren't affordable or practical. However, in the final lead-up to a big event that you're focusing on, a massage can give you a bit of a boost and make you feel 'pro'. Also, a regular – say, monthly – appointment with an experienced soft tissue therapist can be useful as a body MOT and can help identify areas of tightness or concern, which you can then work on yourself.

COMPRESS

Compression clothing has become incredibly popular with athletes of all levels and, although the performance gains during activity are still debatable, there's a fair amount of evidence for their role in aiding recovery post-exercise. The earliest manifestation of compression clothing was in a clinical environment. Post-op, patients wearing tights or socks were found to have improved blood flow and a reduced risk of venous thrombosis (blood clots). In more recent times, this ability to help prevent clots has been used to manufacturer in-flight socks that help lower the risk of deep vein thrombosis during long-haul travel. From a post-exercise recovery perspective, it appears that the benefits are due to enhanced venous return and circulation, but the exact mechanisms aren't fully understood. It's important that you do some research when buying compression clothing and look for clinical graded products that offer graduated compression. Sizing is also very important – unsurprisingly, they have to be tight. A bit like massage, it's possible that the main benefits of compression may be psychosomatic but that's not necessarily a bad thing. It's not a big hassle to put some on post-ride, especially if you have a long drive home, and they're certainly not going to do any harm.

RIDE

As we discussed in Chapter 4, a recovery ride the day after a long or hard ride or race can reduce the sensations of 'stiffening up' and DOMS. However, you have to follow the ride guidelines strictly and it has to be super easy. Stray out of Zone 1 or put significant torque through your cranks and you won't be facilitating recovery, you'll just be accumulating junk miles and fatigue. If you're heading out for a recovery ride, leave your ego behind and, if you don't think you'll be able to handle being overtaken by nearly all other riders, do the session indoors or opt for some sofa time.

SLEEP

All mammals and birds sleep. Deprive a rat in a laboratory of sleep and it'll soon start behaving strangely and gaining fat, and will eventually die. However, for such an essential part of our existence, the exact mechanisms and purpose of sleep are still not fully understood. Simple R&R for the body is not a satisfactory explanation and studies have shown that one of the things sleep deprivation does not impair is physical work capacity and is much more of a cerebral activity. This means if you suffer from poor sleep due to pre-event nerves, your physical performance shouldn't be significantly reduced. However, long-term poor or reduced sleep will result in diminished mental performance and an increase in the body's stress hormone cortisol. This will impact on your ability both to train and to recover. If you're constantly having to get up super early to fit in your training, this will have a negative effect and you should consider revising your training plan and expectations. Additionally, as mentioned earlier in the chapter, disturbed sleep can be a sign of non-functional overreaching.

> 'A recovery day has to be just that and, if you do ride, it has to be super easy. You're barely pressing on the pedals. A lot of riders don't understand this. I've met friends for a ride, have said I'm on a recovery ride and they're surprised how seriously I take riding easy!'
>
> **TIFFANY CROMWELL**, CANYON/SRAM

As an athlete, quality sleep is vital, so do everything you can to optimise it.

- Use the bedroom only for sleeping and sex. Associate the bedroom with relaxation. Get rid of the TV.
- Don't train hard less than 2 hours before sleeping.
- Chill out with some stretching, yoga or meditation before going to bed.
- Avoid/reduce caffeine, nicotine and alcohol before bedtime. Drink warm milk as it contains the natural sleepy chemical tryptophan.
- Avoid arguments, work-related material, discussion of/dwelling on problems near bedtime. Have a cut-off time and stick to it.
- Practise muscle relaxation and mindfulness techniques. There are number of audio guides available.
- Go to bed only when sleepy. Don't try to force it until a regular sleep pattern is resumed.
- If unable to sleep, get up. Write down thoughts in a sleep diary (if a problem

keeps you awake or you remember something you need to do/have forgotten to do, write it down, then forget about it until morning – you have written your reminder).

- Keep the bedroom at a comfortable, well-aired temperature. Check that your pillows and bed linen are comfortable and if not, change them.
- Get up at a regular time, even if still sleepy, and avoid napping. This will aid in the return of a normal sleep rhythm.
- Don't lie in bed worrying that you cannot sleep. This will overstimulate the brain to further awakening. Do not watch the clock, as this encourages a stress response. Not everybody needs 8 hours – give your body the chance and it'll find its own perfect sleep pattern.

▼ If fitting in your training means losing sleep, you need to reassess your training.

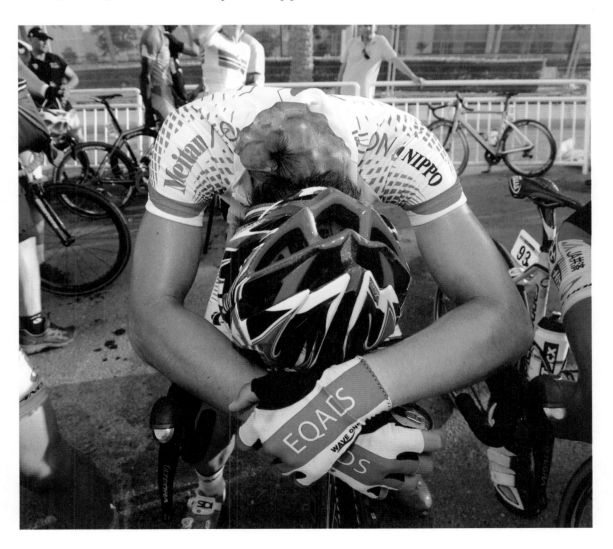

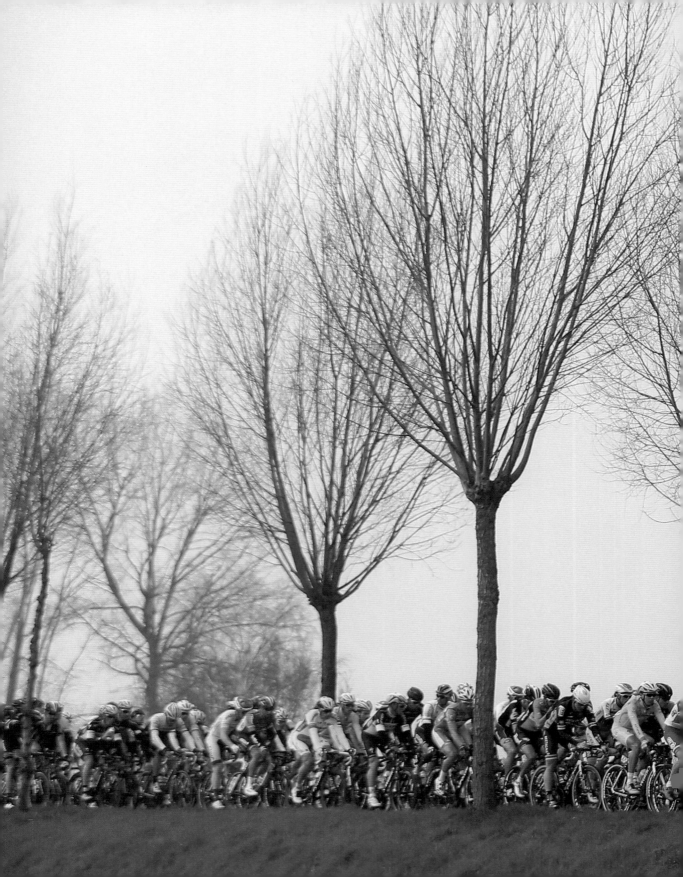

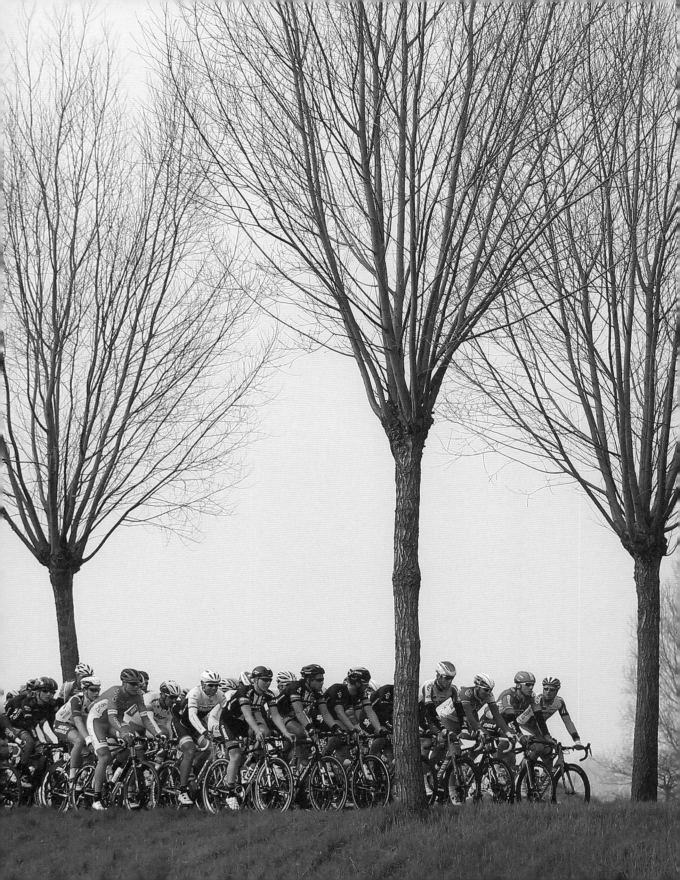

Recovery techniques to avoid

There are a couple of recovery measures that, although used by some riders and even recommended by some coaches, you should avoid.

ICE BATHS

Ice baths are often touted as being beneficial for recovery but their value for cyclists is very limited. Players of contact sports use them to reduce bruising and, for this, they're very effective. The reason you shouldn't be subjecting yourself to ice baths, aside from them being extremely unpleasant after a long winter ride, is that you don't want to reduce the body's inflammation response to training. It's the healing and recovery from this response that leads your muscles to become stronger and thus to performance gains. The only situation when an ice bath may be beneficial is during a multi-day event, where you wouldn't want muscle soreness to inhibit your performance the next day. However, with the research jury still out on the benefits for endurance recovery and it not being used by pro teams on Grand Tours, you should save the ice cubes for your post-ride shake.

PAINKILLERS

Similarly, popping a few painkillers during or after a hard ride to prevent soreness the next day may seem like a good idea. As mentioned above with regard to ice baths, trying to alleviate the inflammatory process can result in reduced training gains. Studies at Ironman Brazil and the Western States 100 Mile Trail Race showed no benefits of taking ibuprofen with regard to perceived discomfort either during or after the events. However, there are also potential health implications. Worryingly, the Western States study showed signs of kidney impairment and endotoxemia (bacteria leaking from the colon into the bloodstream), and also higher levels of tissue inflammation. Painkillers should only be taken under doctor's orders for a specific injury. Research has also shown that risks of hyponatremia (dilution of body salts leading to potential death) in endurance athletes increases significantly when taking painkillers, so it's not worth the risk.

Multi-day rides

It's often said of Grand Tours that it isn't the best rider who wins, it's the best recoverer, and if you're taking on the challenge of a multi-day event, doing everything you can to maximise recovery is your number one priority. Everything that we've previously covered regarding pacing, fuelling and hydration are even more pertinent for multi-day events, as any mistakes you make will be compounded day on day. In the same way that, on a single day ride, you're not eating and drinking for that moment but for 15–20km (9–12 miles) down the road, everything you do on a multi-day ride will impact on subsequent days. Post-ride recovery techniques will definitely help but what

TO SHAVE OR NOT TO SHAVE

Making massage and the treatment of road rash easier are two of the most common reasons given for cyclists, both male and female, shaving their legs. There's no doubt that smooth legs are more pleasant to massage – there's less

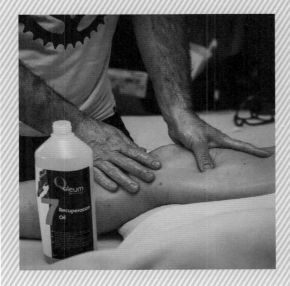

hair pulling and you're not as likely to suffer from folliculitis – but a few massage therapists have confirmed that unless the legs are freshly shaven, stubble makes it like massaging a cactus. Also, if you're not having regular massage, that reason just doesn't quite stack up. Treating road rash is also far easier with shaved legs. You can clean the wound more effectively and dressings stay put and aren't excruciating to remove. However, how many times do you fall off and have to treat road rash?

Fortunately, if you do like to keep your legs smooth, the wind tunnel has come to your rescue. We already mentioned in Chapter 1 that Specialized ran a series of tests and, using six riders with varying degrees of pre-shave hairiness, found an average saving of 50 seconds over 40km (25 miles). To put that in perspective, it's a similar saving to upgrading a traditional round-tubed bike to a highly aerodynamic design.

However, if we're honest, we shave our legs because it identifies us as cyclists and, when you're in good shape and have a bit of a tan, it looks great.

▲ Shaved legs won't make you a great cyclist but they're definitely part of the image!

you do on the bike will have the biggest impact on how you'll perform the next day.

If you're preparing for a multi-day event, your training should reflect this and you should plan a number of 2–3-day blocks where you ride consecutive days that mirror the demands of your event. This will give you the opportunity to test your pacing and fuelling strategies and see if you need to tweak them. It's not necessary to do back-to-back long days every week, which due to the fatigue that this would develop, would in fact be counterproductive. However, putting some in at the end of a 3-week build will be a good test of how your body responds and, with the build weeks in your legs, mimics the feeling of a longer multi-day event well. Also, as you'll have an easier recovery week afterwards, if it doesn't quite go to plan you won't be impacting on important future training sessions.

Many riders find that if they pace, fuel and recover well during multi-day events, they seem to become stronger as the ride goes on and this 'riding into form' is a commonly observed phenomenon. Obviously, this might just be relative to the riders around you becoming weaker or because other stressors in your life such as work and family are removed but, whatever the reason, enjoy it!

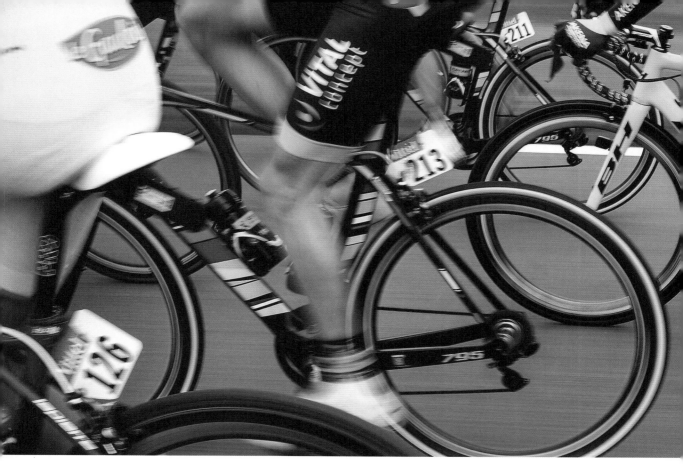

How to improve your cycling performance

Balance recovery and training

Training smart and effectively isn't about simply ticking off training sessions each week. If you're not allowing adequate recovery from your training and racing, you're compromising your gains and potentially risking illness and injury. For non-full-time riders, non-cycling factors have to be considered in your training load and if, for example, work is especially busy or family life demanding, it might be necessary to back off training and place more of an emphasis on recovery.

Functional vs Non-Functional Overreaching

At the end of a 3-week build period or even after an especially tough session, you're going to feel tired and that's okay. You can expect to see a slight dip in your performance but, with recovery, you adapt and bounce back stronger. This functional overreaching is the basis of any structured training plan. However, if you have a 'more is more' mindset and just keep piling on the training without adequate recovery, there's no bounce back, gains stall and performance will start to fall off. If this occurs, you are in a state of non-functional overreaching.

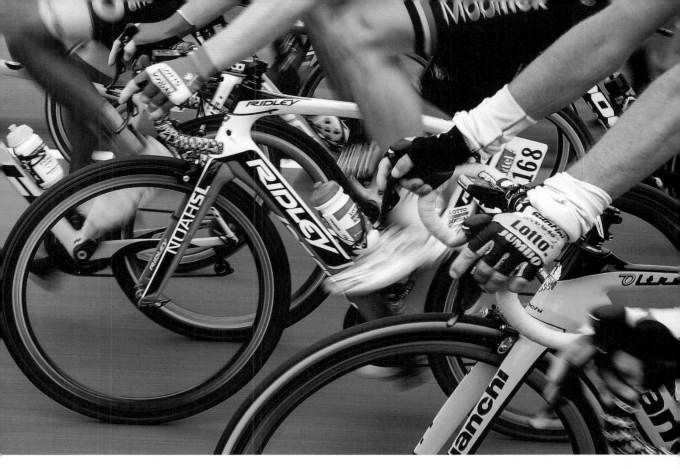

Watch for the signs

There are a number of warning signs of non-functional overreaching and if you start exhibiting more than a couple on consecutive days, you should take action. The key signs to look for are a drop in performance, persistent illness, change in resting heart rate, unexpected sudden or extreme weight loss, poor or interrupted sleep, excessive muscle soreness and irritability or poor mood.

Rest, recovery and time off

Rest and recovery has to be as structured as training and factored into your plan. You should have at least one full rest day each week; a recovery week, with significantly reduced training load, every fourth week; and ideally you should have 4–6 weeks off from structured training at the start of the off season each year.

Maximise rest and recovery

There are a number of techniques that you can use to maximise your recovery after each ride and on rest days. You won't be able to do all of them all of the time but, at the very least, prioritise always having a good cool-down, your post-ride nutrition and doing everything you can to get enough quality sleep each night.

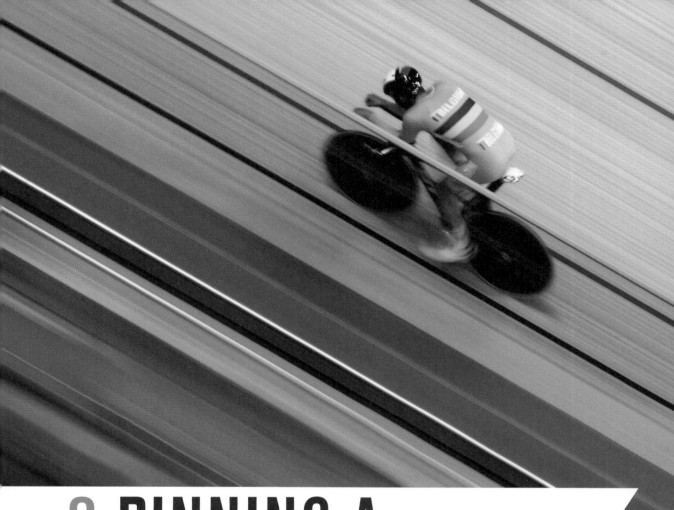

8 PINNING A NUMBER ON

WHEN YOU'VE PUT IN THE TRAINING, NOTHING BEATS PINNING A NUMBER ON AND SEEING HOW YOU FARE AGAINST OTHER RIDERS. THIS CHAPTER LOOKS AT SOME OF THE DIFFERENT DISCIPLINES OF CYCLE SPORT, THEIR DEMANDS AND WHY YOU SHOULD CONSIDER GIVING THEM A GO.

'Cycling isn't a game, it's a sport. Tough, hard and unpitying, and it requires great sacrifices. One plays football, or tennis, or hockey. One doesn't play at cycling.'

JEAN DE GRIBALDY (1922–1987), CYCLING PRO AND LEGENDARY DIRECTEUR SPORTIF

SPORTIVES AND GRAN FONDOS are a fairly recent phenomenon, with the first L'Étape du Tour only taking place in 1993. There is no doubt that these mass participation events have reinvigorated cycling in many countries, providing accessible, enjoyable and challenging events for all levels of cyclists. For many riders, especially with the line between sportives and racing becoming blurred by events such as the UCI Gran Fondo World Championships, they provide more than enough motivation to train for and a competitive outlet. At multi-day events such as the Haute Route, the top-ranking riders aren't far from professional level and, with prize money on offer at some Gran Fondos for the fastest finishers, some take them extremely seriously. Many sportives follow the professional racing calendar and allow non-professional riders to tackle the same roads as their heroes and heroines. Completing an event such as the L'Étape du Tour, the Ronde van Vlaanderen sportive or the Tour of the Battenkill Gran Fondo is a great achievement and a massively worthwhile training goal.

However, as a teak-hard gnarled old racer once said to me on the start line of one of the UK's most challenging sportives, the Fred Whitton: 'It'll be a tough day out but if the number's on your handlebars, it's not a real race. For that real buzz, you've got to pin a number on your back.'

'I have to enjoy racing as I don't really enjoy training! Even with all the nerves and pressure, I know I'd miss it if I didn't do it.'
KATIE ARCHIBALD, GREAT BRITAIN CYCLING TEAM

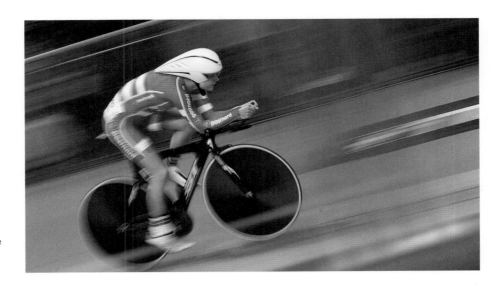

◄ Pin the number on, put on your game face and put all the hard training to the test.

With racing licences, categories and rankings to try to get your head round, getting into racing can appear slightly daunting and intimidating. However, by joining your local cycling club and getting in touch with your national governing body, you'll find plenty of people to guide you through the process. Many riders worry that they may not be fit enough or possess the skills necessary for racing. However, if you can complete a typical sportive, you definitely have the endurance, and it's by racing and tuning your training to it that you'll develop the higher end fitness, skills and race craft.

Most forms of racing allow you to compete on a weekly basis and this is good for a number of reasons. As the cost of entry is usually fairly low compared to a big sportive or Gran Fondo, and you have another go next week, you can afford to experiment and make a few mistakes. You'll have an excellent measure of your progress and it's generally easier to motivate yourself to go and race than to do another gruelling session on the turbo and you're guaranteed a decent workout. Finally, by competing more, rather than banking all of your training and effort towards one or two events each year, you'll become more comfortable with competition and far less likely to suffer from nerves when a big event does come around.

'You'll get a lot of riders who might set themselves the goal of just one big event each year and this can create a lot of pressure. They'll do their training but don't practise event day. I was coaching a rider who was focused on the Marmotte and I got him to do a number of local sportives and races, tapering and peaking for a couple of them and treating them as dry runs for the big day. It really helped and meant he didn't freeze or panic before the Marmotte as all of his processes were rehearsed and in place.' **DEAN DOWNING**, EX-PRO, FORMER BRITISH CIRCUIT RACE CHAMPION AND NOW COACH

Road and circuit

Road racing, typified for most people by the Tour de France, sees the professionals tackling distances of 250km (155 miles) or more in a single-day race or, in the case of stage races and the Grand Tours, racing for multiple days and up to three weeks. At lower levels of the sport, races tend to be far shorter, typically covering 50–100km (31–62 miles) depending on age, sex and level of the event. Also, for amateur events, the roads won't necessarily be fully closed to traffic and it's essential to be aware of whether this is the case. Although road racing is extremely exciting to take part in, if you're just getting into racing, circuit races are a better place to start.

Circuit races take place on closed circuits, utilising dedicated tracks, motor circuits or even aerodromes, and provide a great way to get into racing. The size of the field is determined by the circuit but, with races normally categorised based on age, sex and current ranking, you can expect to be up against riders of a similar ability to yourself. Races are over a set number of laps, typically last for 45–60 minutes and, during the

▶ Shoulder to shoulder, there are few things which beat the thrill of bunch racing.

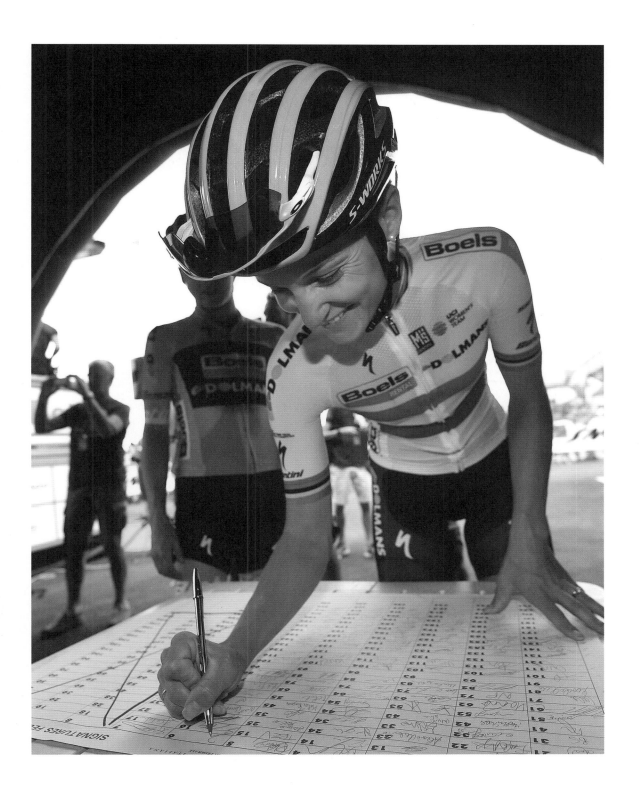

season, often follow a league structure with midweek evening and weekend racing. This style of racing provides the perfect environment to develop your racing skills and fitness as you can race every week. With the circuits usually being relatively short, it doesn't matter if you get dropped by the bunch as you won't have far to ride to the finish on your own. You can set yourself your own goals. At first you might aim simply not to be lapped but, a few weeks into the season, your objective would be to finish in the bunch. You might then set yourself the goal of getting in a break or trying to be near the front to contest the sprint. Eventually, as the season wears on and your skills and fitness develop, you could find yourself earning ranking points, contesting the win and moving up the racing categories.

If you come from a sportive or triathlon background and are a strong rider, you might find, when racing at the entry level categories, that you're able simply to ride off the front, rapidly accumulate ranking points and quickly move up the rankings. However, as tempting as this may be, it can be wise for your long-term racing career to hold back and spend at least a few races sitting in the bunch. Successful and safe racing isn't just about having the biggest engine – good bunch and handling skills are just as important. It's far better to learn these skills and become comfortable in a bunch at a lower level of racing than to suddenly find yourself out of your depth in a faster-moving higher category field.

Whereas you'll typically ride a sportive at a relatively consistent intensity, a circuit race demands repeated micro-sprints as the bunch eases and slows down into corners and then accelerates hard out of them. The further you are down the bunch, the more pronounced this effect and this is a good reason to quickly develop good bunch-riding skills and to position yourself near the front. Making a break also demands the ability to put in a hard, near maximal effort, then to dial it back slightly to hold your gap and then

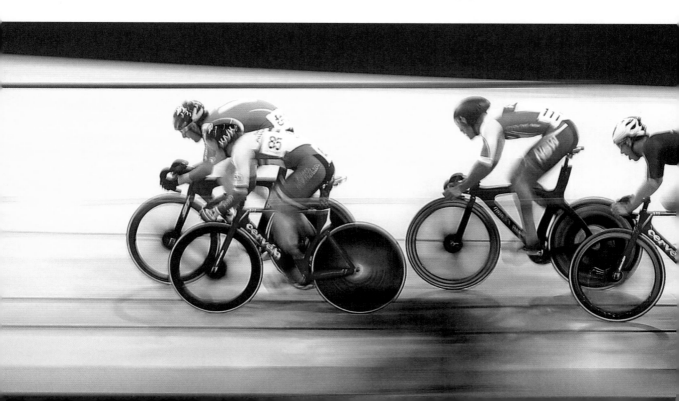

to either be able to time trial to the finish if you're solo or work with your breakaway companions and contest the final sprint. However, most circuit races come down to a bunch sprint so having a decent finishing kick is essential. During the off season, you should focus on building a solid endurance base and your ability to hold prolonged efforts of threshold intensity. However, although this fitness will probably allow you to hang in the bunch, to be competitive you'll need, as you go into pre-season, to work on VO2 (Zone 5), anaerobic capacity (Zone 6) and top-end 10–20-second sprint efforts.

Good bunch and general bike handling skills are essential, along with an awareness and understanding of communication and general group-riding etiquette. The best way to acquire the skills and knowledge is to join and ride with your local cycling club. Remember, everyone was a novice at some point so if you see something you don't understand, don't be afraid to ask.

Track

Track cycling takes place on a purpose-built velodrome. Either indoors or outdoors, the length, geometry, surface and steepness of the banking of the track can vary significantly from venue to venue. The tracks that you'll see used for the Olympics, World Championships and World Cup will be wooden, 250m (820ft) in length and have banking on the bends of around 40 degrees. However, some older outdoor tracks can be 450m (1,476ft) long and have banking as shallow as 10 degrees. Bikes used on the track are fixed gear and don't have brakes. Although this may seem terrifying, it actually makes racing safer as it means that riders in front of you can't slow up suddenly. Picking the right gear to use is a crucial part of track racing and can often be

▼ Fixed gear, no brakes, steep banking and high speeds, what's not to love about track racing!

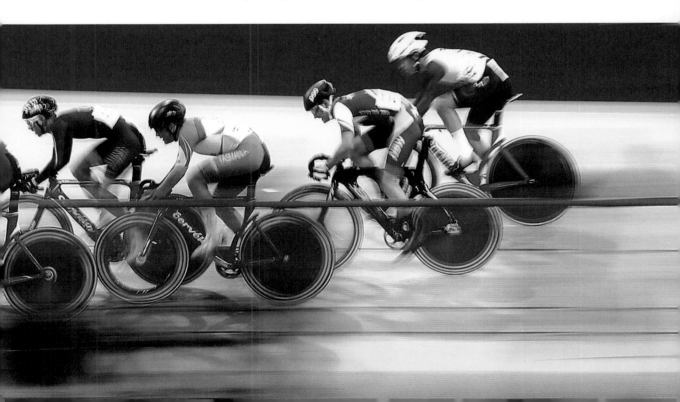

the difference between winning and losing. Too big and you'll struggle to get moving or respond to attacks, too small and you'll spin out before hitting top speed.

Track cycling is split into sprint and endurance events. The sprint events, including match sprinting, 500m/kilo time trial, team sprint and keirin, are extremely specialised. Track sprinters will spend as much time in the gym as they do cycling, if not more. If you're reading this book and come from a road riding background, the endurance events will be what you'll probably gravitate towards.

Even if you're an experienced road rider, most velodromes insist on you going through an accreditation process before racing on the track. The exact process varies from track to track but during it you'll learn the essential skills needed to ride safely on the track. Once you've completed your accreditation, the next stage is to attend a number of structured quality training (SQT) sessions. During these sessions, you'll further develop your track cycling skills, build track-specific fitness and take part in some mock races.

Your first experience of racing on the track will probably be at a track league type event. With a number of different groups, based on age, sex and ability, during the course of an evening meet you'll usually take part in 4–6 different races. These might include the following:

SCRATCH RACE This is probably the simplest bunch race on the track, where the first rider over the line at the end of the set number of laps, typically between 12 and 60 on a 250m (820ft) track, takes the win. It's always a tactical battle between riders with a strong sprint, who'll want it to stay together until the end, and the more endurance-leaning riders, who'll try to break away and take a lap.

COURSE DES PRIMES This is always popular at track leagues and, over a relatively short race, usually around 12 laps, riders contest a sprint every lap for prizes, money or league points. Often the final sprint offers bonus points or a special prize.

ELIMINATION RACE OR DEVIL TAKE THE HINDMOST In this race, every lap or every two laps, the last rider to cross the line is eliminated. This continues until there are just two riders (or a predetermined small number of riders) left, who contest the final sprint.

POINTS RACE Most track leagues finish with a points race. Over a set number of laps, usually 40–60, riders accumulate points at sprints every 5–10 laps. The first rider to cross the line at the end of a sprint lap is awarded 5 points, with 4 points to the second rider, 3 to the third, 2 to the fourth and 1 point to the fifth. The big prize comes for gaining a lap on the field, which is worth 20 points – the equivalent of winning four sprints. Similarly, losing a lap will cost you 20 points. As well as testing you physically, keeping track of your position in a points race is a real mental challenge, especially if there isn't an electronic scoreboard. A variation of the points race is the Madison, where pairs of riders compete. While one rider in the pair is 'active' in the race, the other circles high on the track before being relayed into the action by his or her

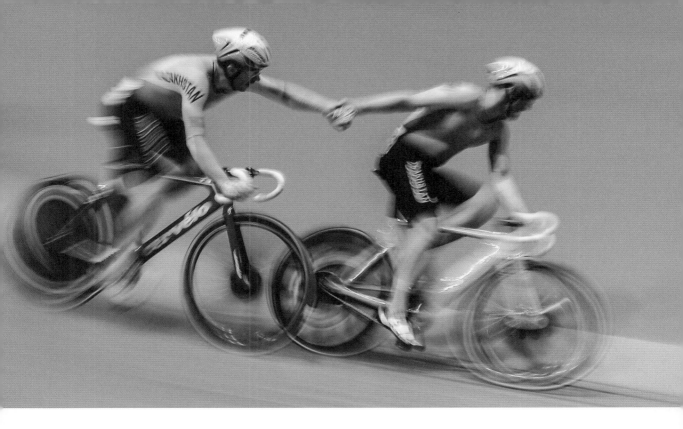

partner, using a hand-sling. A thrilling form of racing to take part in and spectate, the Madison is probably the ultimate test of track skill and fitness.

There are a number of other events and variations that you may encounter during a track league season but the common themes for bunch racing on the track are hard riding and multiple sprints.

Along with the bunch events, as an endurance rider you might find yourself drawn to the individual pursuit. Because of only two riders competing at a time and the need for starting gates, it's not an event that you get to ride very often and tends only to feature at championship meets. Competing over 2–4km (1¼–2½ miles) depending on age and sex, it's simply a head to head with another rider starting opposite you on the track. You'll usually ride a qualifying heat, which is effectively a time trial, and then the two fastest riders will race for gold and silver and the third and fourth fastest for the bronze. In the medal rounds you can win by catching your opponent, which ends the race. The individual pursuit, although appearing so simple, is frustratingly but addictively complex. Gear selection, start technique, pacing, racing line and aerodynamics all have to be spot on to achieve the perfect ride.

If you can find three like-minded friends, you could also try the team pursuit. Although classed as an endurance event, the speeds now ridden in the team pursuit at the highest level, averaging well over 60kph (37mph) from a standing start, are blurring the line between sprint and endurance. At any level, the team pursuit involves

½–2 lap maximal efforts on the front, perfectly executed changes, riding within inches of the wheel in front and then attempting to recover while still riding at or above your threshold.

Predominately racing track myself, I'm probably slightly biased, but if you want to take your cycling to the next level, make riding and racing on the track a priority. It's no coincidence that one of the cornerstones of the Great Britain Cycling Team's development programme is track cycling, and specifically developing the skills and fitness for the Madison. It really does provide young riders (and not-so-young riders) with a brilliant grounding that's applicable to all branches of cycle sport. The high cadences involved develop a silky-smooth pedal stroke that'll translate brilliantly to the road, as will the bunch riding and bike handling skills. If you have an indoor velodrome conveniently close, it's a brilliant way to stay sharp during the winter.

Track cycling is all about the ability to sprint, sprint and sprint again. You don't necessarily have to possess the fastest sprint or be able to produce the highest peak wattage but, having already battled four or five sprints and covered attacks deep into a points race, you need to be able to find another kick to contest the finish. Sessions such as the Tabata workout are ideal for developing this ability and performing them on rollers is great for working on the high cadences required.

Cyclo-cross

Cyclo-cross races are usually held in parkland and open spaces, often in urban areas. The courses are usually about a mile in length, involving a mixture of surfaces and terrain. They'll often be steep climbs, steps, hurdles or thick mud, forcing you off your bike and into a run. Being able to fluidly change from riding to running and back again without losing speed is one of the key skills of cyclo-cross. Races typically last for up to an hour plus one lap – a bell is rung at the end of the set time to signify the final lap. Junior, veteran and novice events are usually shorter. Although there are sometimes some technical sections, the degree of difficulty is nowhere near that experienced in a mountain bike race. A good cyclo-cross course will keep the racing fast, furious, and have you on and off your bike and at your limit for the whole race.

At first glance, a cross bike looks pretty much like a road bike, but there are a few subtle differences. The most obvious are the tyres, which, although much skinnier than on a mountain bike, are still knobbly for better off-road grip. Tubular tyres are favoured by many cyclo-cross racers as they allow riders to run super low pressures for better grip but with less chance of pinch flats. Top riders will have multiple wheelsets with different tubes glued on for a range of conditions and will agonise over the optimal tyre pressure for the day. Tubeless tyres now offer a great compromise if your budget doesn't quite stretch to multiple wheelsets. You can still run low pressures but changing tyres to suit the course isn't too much of a hassle. Cross bikes traditionally had cantilever brakes, but now disc brakes have become standard. Many cross riders will fit additional bar-top brake levers as much of the riding, especially more technical sections, is done with the hands on the tops. Gearing is following the trend in mountain biking with single chainring set-ups and a wide-ranging cassette. Pedals are dual-sided mountain biking pedals, allowing fast mud clearing, easy re-engagement and for the rider to use recessed cleats for running.

Most local races will allow you to take part in cyclo-cross on a mountain bike, so if you have one sitting gathering dust in the garage, stick some skinnier tyres on it and give it a go. However, on a cross course, a true cross bike will always be faster and, be warned, it's a highly addictive sport and I can guarantee you'll soon be adding a crosser to your stable. Most top cross riders will have a twin set of race bikes and, if the course is really muddy, will swap bikes at the end of laps. The poor pit crew then have to manically clean the mud-caked bike in time for the next changeover.

Generally taking place during the winter, although summer leagues are becoming more popular, cyclo-cross provides a great way to keep fit and competitive through the off season. Because of the multi-lap format, you're almost guaranteed to find yourself in your own race within the race, battling with the riders around you and the course even if you're not up at the sharp end. Cyclo-cross races are extremely friendly and welcoming and, with races for all ages and abilities, are brilliant for bike-mad families. It's especially good for young riders as there's no traffic to worry about and the bike handling skills you learn from cyclo-cross provide a great foundation for all other areas of cycling.

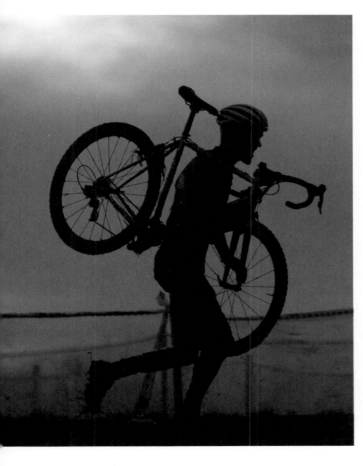

▼ Cyclo-cross is brilliant for fitness, bike handling and getting a racing fix during the winter.

From a training perspective, with races only lasting an hour, if you normally ride sportives you'll have more than enough endurance for cyclo-cross. However, with the constant changes of terrain, pace, dismounts and remounts, the key requirement is being able to maintain an effort at or around FTP/FTHR, but with multiple higher end spikes. A great cyclo-cross-specific workout is a threshold criss-cross Intervals session, but with a 5–10 second sprint at the end of each Zone 5 minute. Don't focus exclusively on fitness, though, as there's a massive skills element to cyclo-cross. If you just try to power your way round a cyclo-cross course, you'll be in for a frustrating experience and will be spending a lot of time on your backside. Head down to some local parkland and spend some time practising dismounts, mounts, running with your bike and riding on loose and slippery surfaces.

THE 3 PEAKS CYCLO-CROSS

The 3 Peaks is a cyclo-cross in name and is ridden on cross bikes but is a distant and meaner cousin to a typical cross race. Held in Yorkshire in the UK every September, it attracts an international field that has included former world champions in both mountain biking and cyclo-cross. It is one of the most challenging and extreme days you can have on a bike and in three attempts I still haven't got it right. Being able to compete in this race is a good enough reason on its own to get a cross bike. The winners take three hours to cover the course while the rest of the field wobble home in up to seven. At 61km (38 miles) in total, encompassing 28km (17½ miles) of road, 33km (20½ miles) of off-road (of which 6–8km/3¾–5 miles is unrideable) and including three of Yorkshire's tallest mountain peaks, this makes for one of the most feared endurance races of the year, taxing both rider and machine. You know a race is tough when it's mandatory to carry a survival bag. The descents off the peaks, particularly the rocky drops off Inglesborough and the stepped slabs of Whernside, would make mountain bikers on full suspension bikes stop and think. The gruelling, almost vertical climbs, with your bike a dead weight on your shoulder, slow even the fleetest-footed mountain goats to a walk.

▼ A cyclo-cross race like no other, the UK's 3 Peaks is a brutal test for both bike and rider alike.

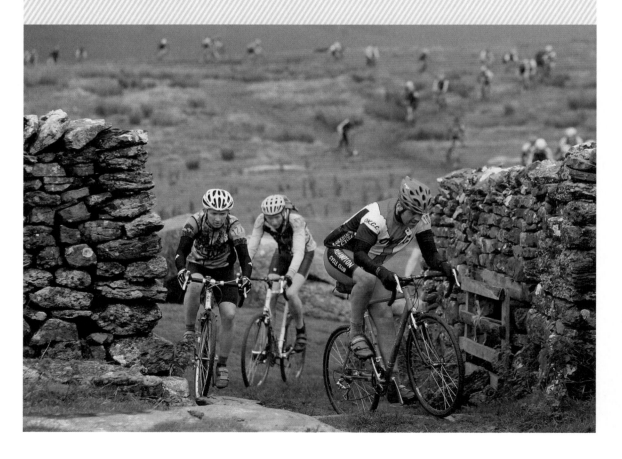

Time trials

Known as the 'race of truth', time trialling tends to evoke a bit of a Marmite reaction from riders – you either love it or hate it. However, no matter what your current level or cycling goals, time trials are a great test of fitness, pacing and mental toughness. Don't be put off by the serious racers in skinsuits, aero helmets and on disc-wheeled stealth bikes. At club events you'll be welcome on any roadworthy bike and remember, it's the clock you're racing against and your performances in previous weeks.

Most cycling clubs will run a weeknight 10-mile (16km), or close to that distance, time trial throughout the summer and into autumn. You don't need to be a club member, they're cheap to enter, you can enter on the night and they're always friendly and inviting. The 18–30-minute effort of a 10-mile TT is an ideal session for boosting your FTP, your sustainable high end level, and, no matter how hard you think you can push yourself in training, you'll always squeeze a bit more out when you pin a number on your back. With weekly events on the same course, you get a regular snapshot of your fitness, which provides great motivation to train. Open events tend to be more competitive and you can often find yourself on the same start list as pros and Olympic champions. They're still friendly and accessible events, though, and with race distance ranging from 10 miles to 24 hours, there's something for everyone.

Don't worry if you don't have a dedicated low-profile TT bike. There will be plenty of riders on standard and modified road bikes, and you're really racing against the course, yourself and the clock. However, there are a few ways to tweak your road bike to make yourself a bit more competitive. For a 10-mile TT, ditch your water bottle and cages. Definitely remove mudguards and there's no need to carry any spares or a saddlebag. Clip-on aerobars can significantly improve your aerodynamics, but don't just blindly stick some on – a road bike's geometry can make it unsuited to clipping on aerobars. You can end up too stretched, with a closed hip angle and, although you may be more aero, your power output might be severely compromised. Fitting a shorter stem and moving your saddle forward on the rails, effectively increasing the steepness, can help to correct this issue, but don't forget you'll probably have to raise your saddle too. Look to minimise your frontal profile, paying particular attention to your shoulders and elbows. Most riders will gain from moving their elbows in but less so if you have particularly broad shoulders. Aim to have your elbows back under your shoulders and not too far forwards. Use a full-length mirror and a home trainer to check your position, make any necessary adjustments, and then see how it feels to ride for 10 minutes at TT effort. There's often a compromise between aerodynamics and power output and you'll need to assess whether you'll be able to train yourself to get used to your new position. The key thing if you do make any changes to your position, especially using clip-ons, is that you practise using them in training. There's no point creating a super aero position for yourself if you're unable to hold it or handle your bike while in it.

Along with optimising your riding position, the best-bang-for-your-buck aero gains are to be had from a decent skinsuit, overshoes and potentially an aero helmet. The first two are no-brainers (make sure you pin your number on neatly, though), but

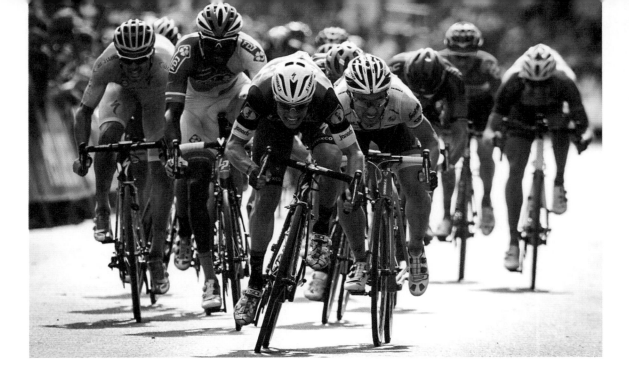

an aero helmet needs a bit more thought. You're looking to obtain a smooth transition from your helmet to your upper back. If you keep your head up when you ride and don't move it around, a long-tailed helmet should work well for you. However, if you tend to move your head about and look down, that tail is just going to stick up in the air and a shorter-tailed helmet or even an aero road helmet would be more appropriate.

Time trials are all about pacing and, especially with 10-mile (16km) and 25-mile (40km) events, it's almost a rite of passage that you'll totally overcook the start of your first few. Power meters really come into their own for pacing time trials but it's important not to be a total slave to your numbers. If you're riding a 10-mile event and know in your last FTP test that you managed to hold 250 watts, this can definitely provide a massively useful pacing metric, but it can also limit you. You might be having a great ride, getting that 'pinning on a number' boost and, as you cross the line, having paced yourself to 250 watts, frustratingly find you haven't totally emptied your tank. Occasionally, try taping over your computer and just riding on feel – you might blow up but, equally, you might get a pleasant surprise. Time trial, prologue and hour record legend Chris Boardman has said the following about pacing time trials, which sums it up brilliantly:

'You will get it wrong but part of the appeal of time trialling is learning from your mistakes and being able to go back the next week, race your previous time and try again. Constantly ask yourself these two questions. How far have I got to go? Is my pace sustainable for that distance? If you answer yes for the second, you're not going hard enough, if no, it's too late and you've overcooked it. You're looking to answer maybe and trying to hover there. I used this simple equation for my whole career and it's served me well.'

▲ Pre-event nerves are normal but, if they're affecting your performance, consider some mental training alongside the physical.

THE PSYCHOLOGY OF PERFORMANCE

One of the major progressive steps of the Great Britain Cycling Team was the appointment of psychiatrist Dr Steve Peters and the realisation of the importance of the mental side of preparation and performance. Like many of the areas we've discussed in this book, we're all individuals and whereas some of us thrive under the pressure, stress and excitement of competition, others crumble and underperform. The sprinter Victoria Pendleton, since retiring, has been especially honest about the work she did with Dr Peters and credits him with much of her success. If you want to further explore his model and way of working, both in sport and everyday life, his book, *The Chimp Paradox*, should definitely be on your reading list.

If you do tend to suffer from event-day nerves, there are a number of practical steps you can take to reduce them.

'Control the controllables' is one of the mantras of the Great Britain Cycling Team and Team Sky. You'll never be able to change the weather or how well your opponents race, but you can make sure that you've trained to the best of your ability, maintained and prepared your bike and equipment well and taken care of pre-event logistics to ensure minimal stress and unnecessary last minute panics. If you've done everything within your control to optimise your performance and execute your plan, that's all you can do.

'I still get really nervous. At the recent World Cup in Manchester I was nervous for the whole week into it and it's a massive stress on your body. It was affecting how I was riding in the days leading up to it and ruining my form. In the end, I had to have a bit of an angry word with myself and stop indulging it. That's not necessarily how to deal with nerves but it worked on that occasion. Everyone gets nervous, even the best riders, it's about finding your own way of coping with them that matters and, for me, when the gun goes off, they disappear.'
KATIE ARCHIBALD, GREAT BRITAIN CYCLING TEAM

Normalising the experience of competition by exposing yourself to it is another effective way to reduce pre-event anxiety. Pros appear so calm and laid-back before a race because they've done it so often. They know their routine, they know the drill so it's no big deal. If you only have a couple of big events each year and have invested huge amounts of time training for them, it's no wonder that you're going to be nervous. Enter lower-key 'B' and 'C' events and, as laid out earlier in the chapter, weekly local races. You'll get used to competition, find and perfect your routine, probably make some mistakes but, when it comes to big events, they won't seem quite so daunting.

'For big races that I knew I could do well at, I'd won before or I knew I was in good form for, then I'd get really nervous. Normally I'm really chatty but I'd becoming really quiet and focused. I'd just get on with making sure everything was right, getting my kit and bike ready. It's part and parcel of competing and you just have to go through your processes.'
DEAN DOWNING, EX-PRO, FORMER BRITISH CIRCUIT RACE CHAMPION AND NOW COACH

Finally, accept that sometimes things just don't go to plan. It could be a puncture, a crash or simply one of those days when your legs just don't fire. Try to take any positives – it might still have been some decent miles in your legs or you might have gained some tactical acumen. Examine if there was anything you might have done differently or better in your preparation or on the day but then move on and don't beat yourself up about it.

Another valuable pacing tip for time trials is to push hardest when you're going slowest. This might sound counter-intuitive but on the slower sections of a TT course, on climbs and into headwinds, you'll take the longest and therefore stand to make up the greatest amount of time. Also, as your speed is lower, drag will have less of an impact so, relative to the extra power you have to put in, you'll go faster. The difference in effort should be quite subtle but significant. For example, if you were riding an out and back course and you knew that coming back it was slightly uphill and into a headwind, you'd hold back a bit on the way out and then push hard into the wind and up the hill. Your overall power target for the ride might be 250 watts so, going out, you'd aim to sit on 240 watts and then, punching back, up it to 260 watts.

Be warned, if you get into time trialling, it can be extremely addictive and you'll soon find yourself chasing the fastest courses and conditions and invariably spending a lot of money on your bike and kit. It's important to remember, however, that although a super aero frame and wheelset will make you faster, 70–80 per cent of drag is down to the rider. Spending some time and money getting your position analysed and optimised would definitely be beneficial. Although wind tunnel time is still prohibitively expensive for most riders, there are now a number of companies who offer affordable velodrome-based analysis.

Training for time trials is all about hard consistent efforts. Sessions such as 20-minute intervals and threshold criss-cross intervals should be your bread and butter, but don't be afraid of throwing in some additional intensity, especially if you're targeting 10-mile events, with 5-minute Zone 5 intervals-type workouts. It's also important that, as much as possible, you train in your racing position. It's not uncommon for riders to lose some power in their time trial position and, as long as this is offset by aero gains, this isn't an issue. However, if this is the case, you should test for FTP in your TT position and set specific TT training zones.

▼ The quest for seconds and a more aero set-up can make time trialling addictively frustrating.

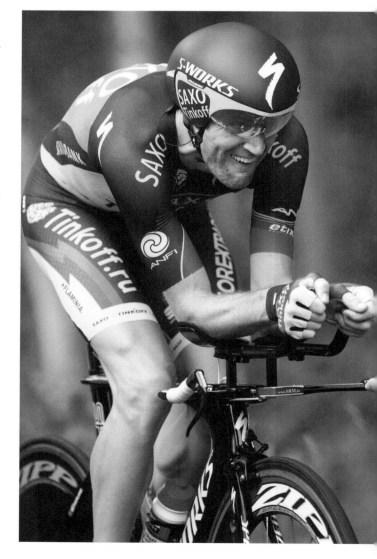

How to improve your cycling performance

Why race?

Sportives and Gran Fondos are great and can be highly competitive, but even if these are your main focus, taking part in regular league-style racing can really up your motivation, fitness and cycling skill set. Racing regularly at low-key local events is the best way to develop your race day routine and will really help minimise nerves for bigger events.

Fitting it in

As we discussed in Chapter 3, you can't taper down every week for a race or you'll never build any level of fitness. The best approach for most forms of racing is to try to schedule an easy day beforehand and then to substitute the race for one of your midweek sessions.

Road and Circuit

Closed circuit racing provides a safe environment to develop your road racing skills and fitness. As with all forms of racing, apart from maybe time trials, it's not necessarily the strongest rider who wins. Focus on trying to develop your bunch riding skills and racing tactics and not just building your engine.

Track

Even if you're a highly experienced and strong road rider, the track is a very different environment and working through your track's accreditation process is essential for making you a safe rider. Make sure you always listen to the coach and don't expect it to be a simple box-ticking exercise.

Cyclo-cross

Good fitness is essential for cyclo-cross but so too are bike handling skills and technique. If you

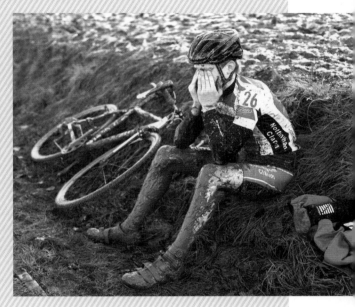

▲ Racing can be tough and unforgiving but, after a hot shower, you'll never regret doing it.

try to rely on strength and power alone, you'll be in for a highly frustrating time. In the lead-up to and during the cross season, try to dedicate a session a week to skills. Set up a loop in your local park or playing field and invite some mates, it'll be a fun and effective workout.

Time trials

Club evening 10-mile (16km) time trials are probably the first experience of racing that many riders have. You don't need a dedicated time trial bike, and you're only really racing yourself and the clock. Make sure, whether you're riding an adapted road bike or a dedicated TT bike, that you've trained in your racing position and, if necessary, have adjusted your training zones.

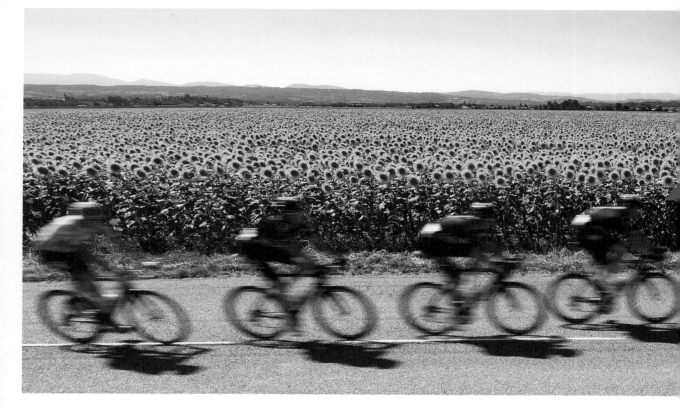

SIGN OFF

HAVING READ THIS BOOK you now have all the tools and knowledge you need to plan and implement a highly effective cycling training plan. Although sports science and its application to performance at the highest level is constantly evolving, the foundations of effective training remain largely unchanged. By ticking these big boxes to the best of your ability, and within the constraints of your life, you'll be harvesting the low-hanging fruit that will undoubtedly have the biggest positive impact on your cycling.

Once you've planned and committed to a training programme, it's essential that you stick to it, follow it consistently, and don't be distracted by or try to incorporate other methodologies or approaches. As cyclists we're constantly bombarded by magazines exposing the latest must-do sessions, wonder supplements or clubmates telling us how they've revolutionized their training. It's tempting to leap from one training bandwagon to the next or to try and do everything but that will only result in inconsistent and ineffective training. Stick to your plan, have confidence in what you're doing and ensure that you're getting all of the basics right.

One of the best bits of advice I ever got was from an old clubmate of mine who

▲ Train hard, train smart, recover well and, above all, enjoy your cycling.

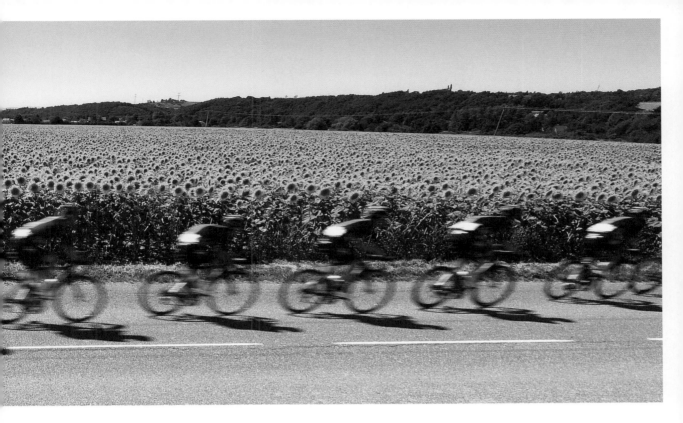

'To me, it doesn't matter whether it's raining or the sun is shining or whatever: as long as I'm riding a bike I know I'm the luckiest guy in the world.' **MARK CAVENDISH**

had been a very successful time trialist and, now into his seventies, was still regularly posting decent times at the club 10-mile events. Knowing that his training time was precious and limited, whenever he got on his bike he'd ask himself what was the goal of the ride, what did it entail and where did it fit in his training plan. Occasionally it would just be going out for a ride simply for enjoyment or to catch up and have a chat with his mates, but he'd be upfront with himself about these rides and make sure they were easy enough not to just build fatigue. Mostly it'd be structured intervals or strict super-easy recovery but there would always be purpose and it would always fit into his plan and complement his other sessions. Apply this mindset to your own riding, always ask yourself why you're doing a ride and what you're wanting to get out of it, and you won't go far wrong.

Above all, though, enjoy your cycling, no matter what your level, and remember, even on those cold and wet winter rides or during gruelling turbo sessions, you're choosing to do it. Take satisfaction in every session you complete, set yourself challenging goals and take pleasure, even if it's under a warm shower afterwards, in every pedal stroke.

Hopefully see you out on the road sometime,

Nikalas Cook

ACKNOWLEDGEMENTS

FIRST OF ALL I'd like to say a big thank-you to Matt and Sarah at Bloomsbury for their patience and invaluable editorial input on this project. Next, I'm extremely grateful to Phil Burt and Nigel Mitchell for their expert advice and assistance. The time given to me by the staff and riders on the Canyon/SRAM pro cycling team, especially Tiffany Cromwell and Hannah Barnes, was incredibly generous. Also the interviews from Phil Gaimon, Katie Archibald and Dean Downing gave brilliant insight into the life and training of top level riders. Finally I'd like to say my biggest thank-you to my wife/longterm bike widow, Lissa. When she said her wedding vows seventeen years ago, I'm not she she realised that it would entail soigneur, pit-crew, psychologist and multiple other cycling related roles supporting my racing. She's put up with an awful lot, including drivetrains in the dishwasher, "taper tantrums" and my leg hairs in the bath, and I'm incredibly grateful to her.

ABOUT THE AUTHOR

NIKALAS COOK is a cycling journalist, coach and rider. He has worked as a consultant with British Cycling for five years, producing training plans and content for their Insight Zone. During that time he has worked closely with key members of the Great Britain Cycling Team, distilling their knowledge and making it applicable to all riders.

He has provided training tips and advice to publications including *Cycling Plus*, *Cycling Weekly* and *220 Triathlon*, where he was their Bike Performance Coach for two years.

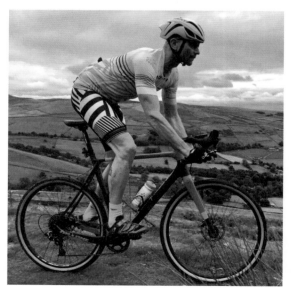

As a coach, he has guided clients through some of the most gruelling cycling challenges including the Étape de Tour, Haute Route, Raid Pyrenees and Tour of Flanders sportive.

As a rider, he's equally at home on road, mountain bike, track or crosser. Notable events he's completed include the seven-day Trans Wales mountain bike stage race, the full distance options of both the Tour of Flanders and Paris Roubaix sportives, the Fred Whitton, the 3 Peaks Cyclo-Cross three times and the Raid Pyrenees. He has also won age-group World Championships in both Long Course Duathlon and Team Pursuit.

INDEX

G

Gaimon, Phil 47, 70, 100, 103, 161, 176
gearing 40
gears, and winter bikes 37, 38
glute trigger point ball 137
goals, training 70
gravel bikes 39
Gribaldy, Jean de 187
group riding 60
groupsets 43
Guarischi, Barbara 93

H

hamstring foam roller 139
heart rate
    and FTHR 48, 49, 53, 59, 63
    monitors 30, 32–4, 47–8
    resting 171
helmets 41–2, 197–8
High Cadence 80, 81, 85, 88, 91, 93, 112
Hoy, Sir Chris 13, 67, 129
hydration 10, 162–4, 167
hyponatremia 162, 163, 182

I

ice baths 182
illness 170, 171
indoor cycling classes 28
indoor trainers 22–5, 45, 105
    midweek workout sessions 109–12
    weekend rides 115–16
indoor training 122
    and FT 58
Indurain, Miguel 65
injury 95, 97

K

Kitchen Sink Pyramid intervals 111
kneeling hip flexor stretch 136

L

Lang, Andreas 31, 34, 52, 74, 92, 137, 169
Lemond, Greg 30, 47
low weight/high rep myth 133–4
lying hamstring stretch 139

M

macro-absorbers 72
maintenance routines 44, 45
marginal gains 7, 8, 9, 28, 41, 44, 67, 164
Martin, Scott 103
massage 177, 183
maximum heart rate 49–50
micro-adjusters 72
midweek workouts 109–12, 122, 126
minimising maximal losses 8–10
minute on/minute off intervals 88, 111, 112, 118, 121, 142
Mitchell, Nigel, *Fuelling the Cycling Revolution* 145
mobility work 131, 134–9, 140, 143
moods, and overtraining/overreaching 173–4
mountain bikes 38–9, 81
mudguards, and winter bikes 38
multi-day rides 182–3

N

nerves, racing 199
nutrition 10, 98, 145
    on the bike 146, 149
    day before a long ride 145–6
    hydration 162–4, 167
    pacing and fuelling 151–2, 167
    pre-ride 146
    pro race-day 150
    and recovery 174–5
    supplements 164–6, 167
    and weight loss 156–61, 167
    and workout sessions 153–5, 158, 160, 167
nutrition post-ride 149

O

Obree, Graeme 22, 169
off the bike training 69–70, 76, 129–30
    mobility work 131, 134–9, 140, 143
    rowing 142, 143
    running 140, 142, 143
    strength work 130–4, 143
    swimming 142
    yoga/Pilates 143

off season 74, 76
    strength sessions 133
    weekend/longer rides 118
    and weight loss/gain 158, 161
off-road cycling 38–9
Omega-3 fats 165
overload 68–9, 70
overreaching *see* overtraining/overreaching
overtraining/overreaching 169, 170–4, 184, 185

P

pacing 10, 47, 167
    and nutrition 151–2
    and time trials 198, 200
painkillers 182
pec stretch 139
peg trigger ball 139
Pendleton, Victoria 67, 199
performance, psychology of 199
Performance Management Chart (PMC) 79–80, 87
Peters, Steve, *Chimp Paradox, The* 199
pigeon pose 137
Pilates 140, 143
planning 101
    a training day 85–6
    weekly sessions 83–5, 94
    a year 74–7
points races 192–3
power meters 30–6, *30*, 45, 101
    and FTP 49, 62, 63
    and time trials 198
    and training 79
    and weight loss 157
pre-event rides 124
professional riders
    and recovery 169
    training diaries 92–3
progressive training 69, 70
protein 146, 160
    post-ride 149
    pro race-day nutrition 150
    and recovery 125
psychology of performance 199
pursuit, individual/team 193–4

Q

quad foam roll 136

R

racing 187–8, 201
  cyclo-cross 194–6
  road/circuit 188–91
  time trials 197–8, 199
  track 192–4
  weekly 90–1
recovery 10, 11, 70, 73, 79, 169, 184, 185
  and cooling down 107
  and effort lengths 119–21
  enhancing 174–9
  and multi-day rides 182–3
  and nutrition 125, 153
  overtraining/overreaching 170–4,
    184–5
  rides 124, 126, 178
  and swimming 142
  techniques to avoid 182
  weeks 84, 85, 89, 94, 98–9
  zone 53
responders 72
rev-outs 104, 106, 112, 121
road races 188–91, 201
rollers (indoor trainer) 22, 23, 25, 105,
  112, 124, 194
rowing 142, 143
running 140, 142

S

saddles/saddle soreness 19–20
Schulze, Julia 98, 131, 156, 170
scratch races 192
set-up *see* fit/set-up
shaving 42, 183
skin-fold test 157
sleep 172–3, 178–9
smart trainers 122
specificity 69–70
sports drinks 163
sprints 34, 121, 192, 194
standing up 176
static bikes 22, 23
Strength Intervals 80, 81, 82, 109,
  112, 118

strength work 130–4, 140, 143
stretching 134, 135–7, 139
supplements 164–6, 167
sweet spot 55, 120
swimming 142, 143

T

Tabata 112, 121, 194
tapering 87–91
tempo (Zone 3) 54
testing, training zones 50–2, 58–9
Threshold Criss-Cross Intervals 110,
  112, 118, 195, 200
threshold (Zone 3) 54, 120
time trials 197–8, 200, 201
tool-assisted self manual therapy
  (TASMT) 134, 135, 136, 137, 139, 143
  and recovery 177
track cycling 192–4, 201
training 10, 65–7, 203
  and altitude 99–100
  blocks 79–82, 85, 95
  carbohydrate-fasted 60, 87, 115,
    125, 152
  for events 73
  fundamentals 68–73, 101
  indoor trainers 22–5, 28–30
  planning a day 85–7
  planning a week 83–5, 94
  planning the year 74–6, 94
  professional diaries 92–3
  recovery weeks 85
  tapering 87–91
  for time trials 200
  winter 11, 37–9
  see also off the bike training;
    training zones; workout sessions
training camps 96, 97–100
Training Stress Score (TSS) 79–80
Training Stress Balance (TSB) 79
training zones 47–50, 53–5
  effort lengths and recoveries 119–21
  problems 59–63
  setting 47–8, 53
trigger point balls 134, 135, 137, 139,
  177
turbo trainers 9, 22, 23, 29, 107, 116

U

urine, and hydration 162, 163,
  164

V

vegetarians/vegans 160
velodromes 191–4
virtual reality 28
Vitamin D 165
VO2 Max (Zone 5) 54–5, 120–1

W

warming up 104–6, 126
weather 115–16
weekend rides 114–16
  and longer rides 117–18
weekly training sessions 83–5, 94
weight loss 125, 167
  rapid 172
What it Takes to Win philosophy 66
wheelsets 43
Wiggins, Sir Bradley 44, 73, 99, 125,
  142
winter
  bikes 37–9
  training 11
  Vitamin D 165
workout sessions 103, 104, 126
  cooling down 107, 126
  midweek 109–12, 122, 126
  and nutrition 153–5, 158, 160
  special 124–5
  warming up 104–6, 126

Y

year planning 74–6, 94
yoga 140, 143

Z

zones *see* training zones

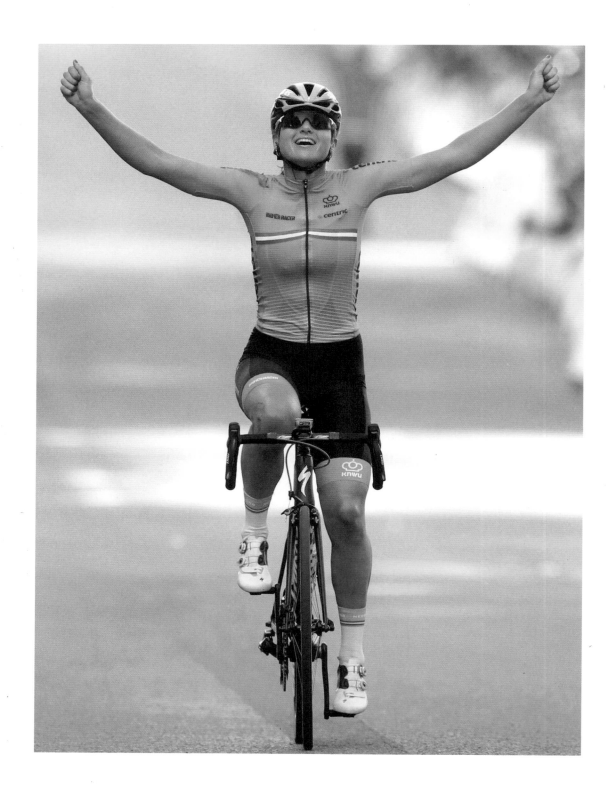